Atlas of Mammographic Positioning

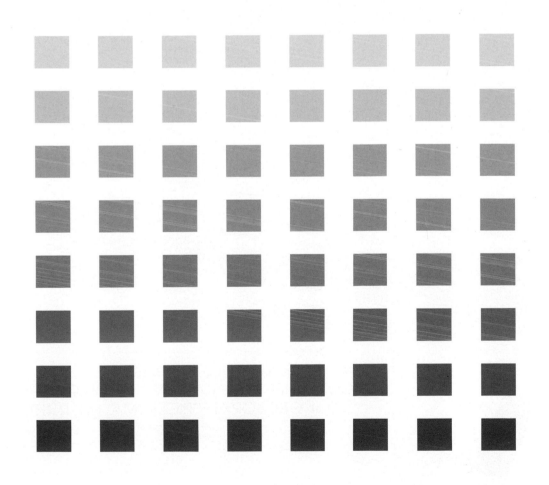

W.B. SAUNDERS COMPANY

A Division of Harcourt Brace & Company

Philadelphia   London   Toronto   Montreal   Sydney   Tokyo

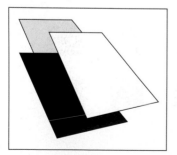

A volume in the Saunders series
CONTEMPORARY IMAGING TECHNIQUES
Editor, GREGORY L. SPICER, MA, MS, RT(R)

LUCINDA K. PRUE, RT(R)(M)

University of Wisconsin Hospital and Clinics
Madison, Wisconsin

Atlas of Mammographic Positioning

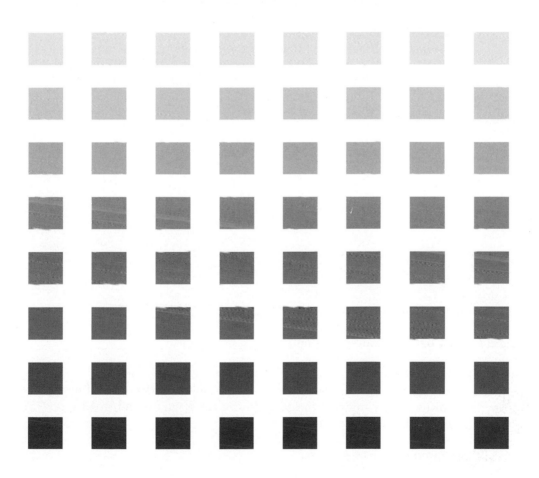

W.B. Saunders Company
A Division of Harcourt Brace & Company

The Curtis Center
Independence Square West
Philadelphia, Pennsylvania 19106

Library of Congress Cataloging-in-Publication Data
Prue, Lucinda K.
     Atlas of mammographic positioning / Lucinda K. Prue,
       p. cm.
     ISBN 0-7216-3683-7
     1. Breast—Radiography—Positioning—Atlases.   I. Title.
     [DNLM: 1. Mammography—methods—atlases. WP 17 P971a]
  RG493.5.R33P78   1993   616.99'24907572—dc20
  DNLM/DLC   92-4980

Atlas of Mammographic Positioning   ISBN 0-7216-3683-7

Printed in the United States of America

Last digit is the print number: 9 8 7 6 5 4 3 2 1

Foreword

Over the past decade, mammography has come into its own as an important subspecialty of diagnostic radiology. The mammography technologist not only must consistently perform precise and high-quality examinations but must also be able to interact with an anxious patient and help allay her fears. Teamwork between the radiologist and the technologist is essential for accurate diagnosis. Despite this important relationship, most mammography texts are directed exclusively toward the radiologist and the analysis of lesions found on the mammogram. However, an abnormality that has not been imaged will remain undiagnosed no matter how great the skill of the radiologist.

In this text, Ms. Prue has addressed these issues in detail, sharing techniques gathered in over 15 years of working in the field of mammography. Much of her career has been devoted to the pursuit of excellence in mammographic technique and to the dissemination of this information via a multitude of educational channels. She has conducted independent seminars in mammographic technique and positioning at hospitals and clinics throughout the United States.

Written in a common-sense, step-by-step fashion, this text should be of great benefit to any technologist striving for excellence in mammographic imaging with the ultimate goal of saving women's lives.

Kathleen Scanlan, MD
Margaret Fagerholm, MD
Pamela Propack, MD
Frederick Kelcz, MD
Fred Lee, MD

Preface

This book is primarily a pictorial essay of mammographic positioning. Starting with the basic screening views, the book goes step by step through each position. It also covers the modified craniocaudal and lateral views as well as spot compression. There is a large section on difficult-to-position patients. The Eklund modified compression technique is included in this section, as well as information covering preoperative needle localization and clinical breast examination. The latest recommendations from the American College of Radiology for standardization of labeling for the mammogram are also listed. I have included a chapter dealing with preparing patients both mentally and physically for the mammography examination.

I began this project with one goal in mind: to pass along workable positioning techniques. Mammographic positioning has undergone many changes in the past few years. Continuing education by attending seminars or reading pertinent publications is needed to ensure the highest level of knowledge and professionalism.

Today the mammography technologist has been called upon to wear many hats. She (or he) must be an artist, shaping and molding the patient's breast against a rigid, unyielding machine. Mammography can be an emotional and trying experience, particularly for women with breast problems. The technologist has become a teacher and counselor, educating patients to the benefits of routine mammography and breast self-examination, as well as alleviating fear of the unknown.

In the pages to come, I will share mammographic techniques that have been gathered from over 15 years of working in the field of mammography. Some of the information comes from mammography radiologists and technologists as well as educators. All of these professionals have a common goal: to fight breast cancer with all available means.

Acknowledgments

I would like to acknowledge and express my deep appreciation for the cooperation and generous support from everyone involved in this project.

The relationship between a mammography radiologist and technologist is a special one. The radiologists I have had the pleasure to work with have always encouraged me to be my best. Thank you all for allowing me to ask as many questions as I needed to understand the entire picture, for I am sure my questions drove you a little crazy.

A special "thank you" goes out to General Electric Medical and the associates I have come to call friends over the last several years. Working with all of you motivates me to a higher level of professionalism.

I would like to acknowledge Instrumentarium Imaging and thank them for the use of their facility and mammographic equipment pictured in many of the photographs in this book.

All of the patient models that I worked with did a wonderful job, and this book would not have gotten off the ground without them. Everyone worked long hours in sometimes adverse conditions (cold equipment and rooms). I would like to thank my photographer, Mr. David Schuh. The photographs that he brought to this book, which showed step-by-step detail of each position, were done with great professionalism. David, it was a pleasure working with you once again.

Several typists worked on this manuscript and did a wonderful job of organizing my notes.

I would like to acknowledge the W.B. Saunders Company, especially Lisa Biello, the Editor-in-Chief of Health Related Professions, for having the faith in my ability to write this book and for standing behind me through its completion.

In conclusion, I would like to thank my family and friends for the tremendous amount of encouragement given to me through this entire process. None of us were aware of the amount of time that would be needed to complete this project. Thank you for allowing me to be as focused as I have been.

I believe mammographic positioning has evolved to the level it has because technologists have shared their experiences with others. Therefore, I am sharing this with you in the hope that it will be useful to all seeking knowledge in the art of mammographic positioning.

Contents

CHAPTER ONE

Preparing Patients for the Mammography Experience

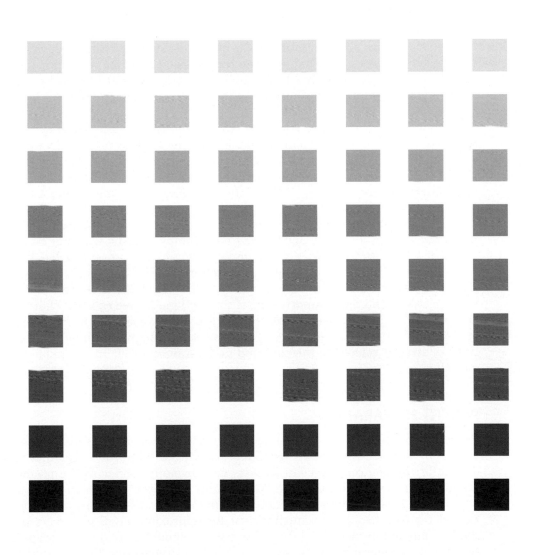

DEALING WITH MISCONCEPTIONS ABOUT MAMMOGRAPHY

Patients have varying ideas of what mammography entails. Some feel that if they take care of their breasts, they will never need to undergo mammography except as problems arise. Others think of undergoing a mammographic study as a torturous event in which their breasts will be locked in a vise and "squashed." They feel that if they do have any lesions in their breasts, the lesions will surely rupture under the pressure of the compression paddle. Many female patients are convinced that the mammography equipment was invented by an unfeeling man who did not care about women's discomfort. The question, then, is how to deal with patients' misconceptions about the mammographic examination.

Many publications available today, including newspapers that carry Ann Landers, have articles that mislead our patients about what having a mammogram involves. Headlines such as "What Doctors Are Doing Wrong" or "Breast Cancer: Was Your Mammogram Really Negative?" cause much fear among women. This fear can be divided into three categories: 1) physical; 2) emotional; and 3) intellectual.

Physical fears are characterized by questions such as "How long will my breasts be compressed? What will the compression feel like, and how much pressure is there going to be? Is this going to hurt, and will I be able to take it? How much radiation exposure will I receive, and will it damage my breast tissue?"

Emotional fears lead to questions and thoughts such as "Are they going to find cancer? Will I be uncomfortable having my breasts touched by another woman? Will the technologist think my breasts are ugly? I am embarrassed to feel so childish and have anxieties such as these. Does the technologist know what she is doing? What if the technologist is a man! I don't know if I can go through with this!"

Intellectual fears make patients ask questions such as "Why are they positioning me in these strange ways? I have lumpy breasts; will they be able to tell if I have cancer? Will the mammography cause cancer? Will I know what to ask? Will I remember what they tell me even if I do ask? How many x-rays can they take on my breast safely? Will they tell me if something is wrong? Lastly and most importantly, if they tell me I have cancer, what is in store for me?" Our patients look to the technologists for answers to these questions. The experience they have during their mammographic examinations is directly related to the care and understanding that the technologists give them.

PATIENT PREPARATION

Preparation begins with scheduling, before the patient arrives at the mammography department. Postmenstrual scheduling will reduce complaints and discomfort during compression. Breasts are normally tender in the premenstrual cycle owing to hormone fluctuation or water retention. Because breasts are least likely to be tender following a patient's menses, the patient should try to schedule the appointment for approximately 5 to 7 days past the last day of her menstrual flow. The patient should be told about preparation for mammography when she schedules it. Preparation for mammography is very simple but often forgotten. If the patient has prepared for her mammography, she will be more relaxed and much easier to work with.

During the examination, the patient will have to remove clothing from the waist up. Wearing a blouse or shirt with either a skirt or a pair of slacks will enable the patient to remain covered on the bottom. In this way, the patient will not feel totally exposed when the gown is partially off.

Patients should also be advised to avoid using powders, deodorants, and perfumes before the examination. These articles are notorious for creating artifacts that may be misdiagnosed as microcalcifications on the x-ray films. If the patient does not use powder or deodorant but overuses perfume to compensate, she may create a problem for the technologist or the other patients she is waiting with by overpowering them with her scent. To create a sense of well-being for the patients and show them consideration for their needs, it is nice for the technologist to supply the dressing room with a hypoallergenic deodorant for patient use after the examination. The technologist may also instruct the patients to bring their own deodorant.

The technologist needs to determine the amount of time to schedule for each mammographic exam when the appointment is first made. It is also necessary to determine if the patient is a paraplegic in a wheelchair or if she has breast implants. For a breast implant patient, 8 to 10 views are needed for a full mammographic study. A patient with a breast lump may require special cone-down or roll views that require additional time. If the patient feels that the technologist is rushing, she may respond accordingly and possibly become uncooperative or even angry. It is important to remember that the more relaxed and comfortable a patient is, the better the mammographic films are going to turn out.

Comparison films, if taken at a different hospital, should be obtained prior to the mammographic exam. The patient should bring them with her or arrange to have them sent to the mammographic facility prior to the appointment. Previous films must always be reviewed with the current study so that the radiologist need not defer his or her final interpretation until the comparison can be made. Previous films, when available to the technologist, sometimes provide important technical information, enabling the technologist to select a more appropriate technical factor. Mammograms taken by other technologists give the technologist a sense of any problems other technologists may have encountered with the patient, such as positioning problems or dense breast tissue. The technologist should note if any extra views, such as cone-down or 90° lateral views, were taken at previous examinations.

GREETING THE PATIENT

When the patient arrives at the reception desk, a warm and congenial welcome sets the stage for a happy and less anxious patient. The registration desk can be a chaotic place to work, with phones ringing and several patients checking in at once. If the patient's first interaction with someone in the x-ray department is totally frenzied, she may become unsettled. An unhappy, frightened patient is less likely to fully cooperate or be helpful in providing needed information. She may also be less responsive to instructions during the examination. A prompt, assisted, and effective registration process will enhance a patient's acceptance and is less likely to annoy or upset the patient.

Having the patient fill out a long registration or information form before any introductions have been made can also upset the patient. This administrative request may suggest to the patient that she will experience impersonal handling by a mechanical functionary. She may feel like a number and not a person. It is important to remember that a helpful manner should prevail throughout the scheduling, registration, and filming processes.

The first task a mammographic technologist has is to introduce herself to the patient and establish rapport. Both first and last names should be used in this introduction. An introduction may be something like, "Good morning, Mrs. Jones, my name is Lucinda Prue, and I will be performing your mammogram today. May I call you Sally, or would you prefer me to use 'Mrs. Jones'?" Many mature patients may think the technologist is being too familiar by using their first names only, so it is important to give them a choice. The technologist should next ask the patient whether she has ever had mammography performed at that facility before. This question provides an excellent beginning to history-taking and will tell the technologist how much of an explanation of mammography is needed. If this is the third or fourth time the patient has been to that facility for a mammogram, it would be redundant to go through the entire procedure with her. If it is the first time, however, the technologist will want to take a little more time in explaining every detail.

EXPLAINING THE PROCEDURE

After the patient has changed clothing but before she has removed the gown for the examination, the technologist should show her the machine that will be used and should carefully explain compression. The technologist may want to tell the patient that compression of the breast helps to separate overlapping breast tissue and reduce radiation exposure. It is important to assure the patient that although compression may be uncomfortable for a few seconds, it should never be painful. The patient should be told to let the technologist know if the procedure becomes painful so that it can be stopped. Mammography involves teamwork. The technologist and the patient are a team, interacting with each other to achieve the best possible images. If the technologist is using an automatic compression paddle, it is helpful to show the patient how firmly it comes down on top of a hand. It is important to familiarize the patient with the sound and the movement of the paddle. The technologist does not want the patient to pull her breast out from under the paddle halfway through compression because the machine is making noise.

It is important to inform the patient about the number of views to be taken. A routine study may sometimes include more than the mediolateral oblique view (MLO) and craniocaudal view (CC). The technologist should make sure that the patient is aware that the procedure begins with 2 to 4 pictures on each breast. Additionally, if the patient is aware that the exam will be tailored to her specific needs, she will not become alarmed if extra views are needed.

After the patient has seen the equipment to be used and has a basic idea of what the technologist is doing, the technologist may want to ask her if she has any questions about the examination itself. The patient will have more confidence in the technologist at this point if given the opportunity to express herself. Once the films have been obtained, the technologist should tell the patient if the films will be shown to a radiologist. The technologist should give the patient an idea of the amount of time needed to develop and show the films. Remember, sometimes a 5- to 10-minute wait may seem like 50 minutes or longer if the patient has a breast problem and is already experiencing anxiety. It is a good idea to keep the patient occupied while the technologist is out of the room; the technologist should give the patient some information to read about breast self-examination or on women's health concerns in the 1990s. In addition, several excellent videotapes on breast self-examination are available. One of these may be a helpful diversion while the patient is waiting for the technologist to return.

As health care professionals, we need to treat each patient with respect and dignity during her mammographic exam, for this is how we want to be treated when we are on the receiving end of this examination. It is imperative to focus all of our energies on each person as an individual, and to address her fears and anxieties, thus making the mammographic experience a positive one.

Ode to a Mammogram—Revisited©
by Louise C. Miller, RT(M)

My doctor had ordered an x-ray of breasts.
Although I was frightened, I knew it was best.

The tech was most gentle and equally kind,
She answered the questions that cluttered my mind.

She told me to practice my breast self-exam;
An exam by my Doctor; they're all part of the plan.

It's not the most fun, though I know it's done right;
If it finds cancer early, she just saved my life.

So I'll tell all my friends, with our fears we can cope;
This tech, this experience, have given me hope.

Copyright by Louise C. Miller, RT(M), 1991

CHAPTER TWO

Basics of Mammography

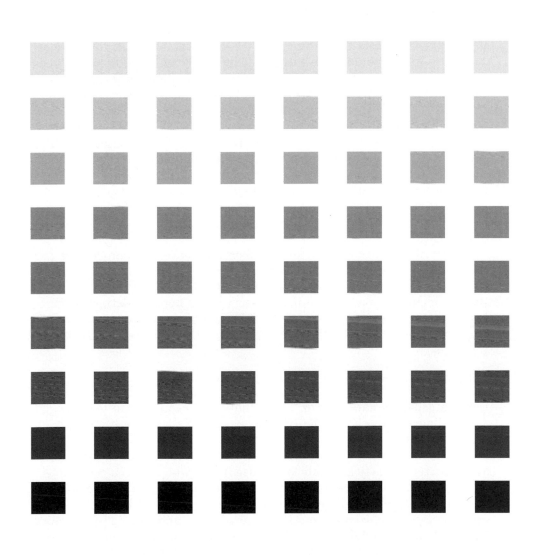

This section covers 1) labeling of the mammogram; 2) compression; 3) standard views for screening, including the craniocaudal view (CC) and the mediolateral oblique view (MLO); and 4) the posterior nipple line (PNL).

STANDARDIZED FILM LABELING

The American College of Radiology (ACR) has recently set forth guidelines for standardized terminology as well as labeling of mammograms. Because mammograms are medical documents, it is important that all films be properly labeled so that they will not be misinterpreted.

The ACR's guidelines are as follows (Fig. 2-1):

1. The film should have a permanent identification label that contains at least the following information: the facility name, the patient's first and last names, a patient identification number (a medical record number, social security number, or date of birth is less desirable), and the date of the examination.
2. Radiopaque markers indicating right or left laterality (R/L) and projection (CC, MLO) should always be placed on top of the cassette holder near the axillary portion of the breast. To eliminate confusion from one facility to another, standardized abbreviations have been developed by the ACR (Table 2-1). Using these abbreviations makes reproducing an extra view for a follow-up on a patient much easier. The technologist strings the abbreviations together to signify the view taken. For example, RCCRM means right craniocaudal upper breast rolled medially. (R = breast being imaged; CC = beam direction; and RM = positioning of breast.)
3. Cassette screen identification is used to identify artifacts or defects on the screen. Numbers may be written on the screen with a permanent marker. Technologists may contact the screen manufacturer for other methods of identification.
4. The technologist performing the mammographic examination should also be identified on the film. The technologist may be identified with initials or a technologist identification number placed either in the designated patient identification area on the film or with radiopaque letters or numbers on the cassette holder itself. A log should be maintained by the radiographic facility of all of its technologists and their identifying initials or numbers.

Other labeling recommendations include the following:

1. Using a separate date sticker. Individual stickers allow the technologist and radiologist to easily identify the past year's examination with an overhead light.
2. Patient identification with a flash card. This way of labeling is permanent and is better than stick-on labels because it is reproducible on copy films.
3. Using self-adhesive stickers to record the technical factors. These stickers have a place for the milliamperage per second (mAs), kilovoltage (kVp), compression force, compressed breast thickness, and degree of obliquity for mediolateral oblique views. Recording this information on films also helps the technologist to reproduce the view in the future.
4. Knowing which machine the examination was performed on, if the facility has more than one mammographic unit. A radiopaque number (U–1, U–2, or I, II) may be placed directly on the cassette holder or buckey.

THE CHARACTERISTICS OF COMPRESSION

The buzzword currently used for "compressed" is "taut." When the breast is compressed until the tissue is taut, the technologist is able to gently tap on the patient's skin without its indenting. Proper compression will 1) hold the breast tissue away from the chest wall; 2) separate overlapping structures; 3) reduce geometric unsharpness; 4) reduce motion unsharpness; 5) reduce scatter radiation; and 6) reduce the radiation dose. If the technologist attempts to be kind and not use as much compression as needed, the results will not benefit the patient. The final film may have poor image quality, and result in a higher patient radiation dose. On the other hand, if the technologist is overly vigorous with compression, the patient may find it painful and decide not to return for periodic screening mammograms. As discussed earlier, in preparing the patient for the mammogram experience, it is important for the technologist to establish rapport with the patient and educate her about compression, including how long it will last and why it is important.

THE MAMMOGRAPHY EQUIPMENT

Whatever name-brand mammography equipment your facility uses, the compression paddle must meet certain criteria. The compression paddle should be ridged with a 90° angle between the posterior and inferior surfaces. If the compression paddle is rounded on the posterior edge, it will not uniformly compress deep breast tissue or hold it firmly in place during the radiation exposure. The edge of the compression paddle that holds the posterior aspect of the breast on the film near the chest wall should be straight rather than rounded. This allows for uniform compression of the breast along the posterior aspect of the film. The compression paddle should be attached to the x-ray machine so that it remains parallel to the plane of the image receptor. A properly designed and applied compression device enables the technologist to maximize the amount of breast tissue imaged in the examination.

TABLE 2-1   Labeling Codes for Positions

Laterality	
Right	R*
Left	L*
Position	
Craniocaudal	CC
Mediolateral oblique	MLO
90° Mediolateral	ML
90° Lateromedial	LM
Magnification	M*
Exaggerated craniocaudal	XCCL
Cleavage	CV
Axillary tail	AT
Tangential	TAN
Roll (laterally)	RL +
(medially)	RM +
Caudocranial (from below)	FB
Lateromedial oblique	LMO
Superolateral to	
inferomedial oblique	SIO
Implant displaced	ID

*used as a prefix before the projection
+used as a suffix after the projection

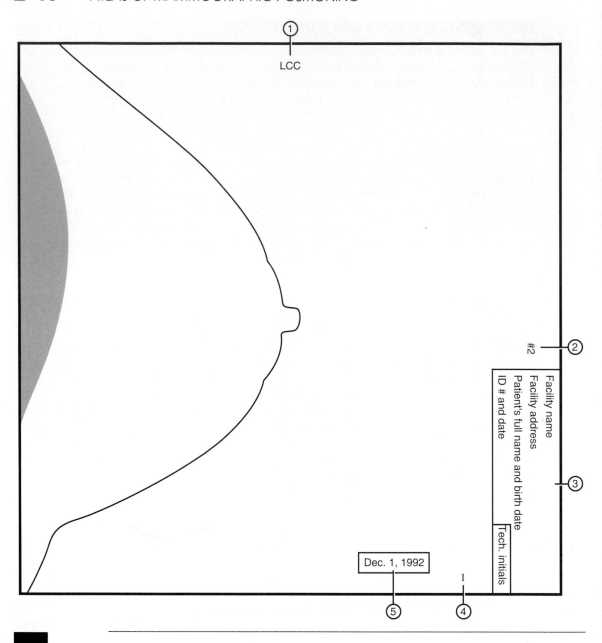

Figure 2-1. Proper film labeling of mammograms. 1: View and laterality; 2: screen number; 3: flash card information (facility name and address, patient's full name and birth date, ID or medical number, date of exam, and technologist's initials); 4: dedicated unit number; 5: date sticker.

Figure 2-2. *A, Top, facing page.* The mobile aspect of the breast for the craniocaudal view lies in the inferior margin. In this figure, the technologist holds the patient's breast so that the inframammary fold (IMF) is in a neutral position.

CRANIOCAUDAL VIEW

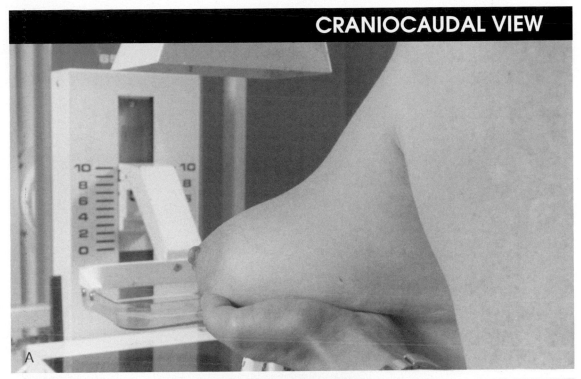

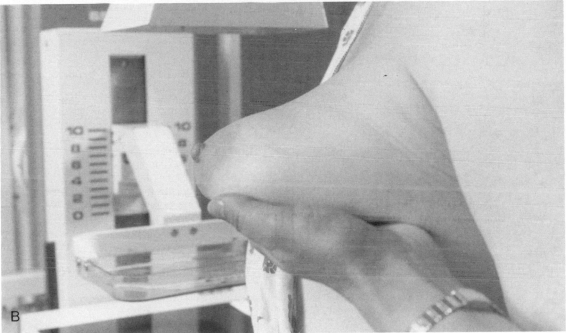

Figure 2-2 *Continued.* **B,** *Bottom.* The technologist may elevate the inframammary fold from 1.5 cm to 7 cm by slowly raising the hand holding the patient's breast. Raising the inframammary fold superiorly toward the fixed border of the breast anteriorly maximizes the amount of breast tissue that can be visualized. The compression paddle will then have less distance to travel across the top of the chest wall; therefore, less breast tissue will be displaced.

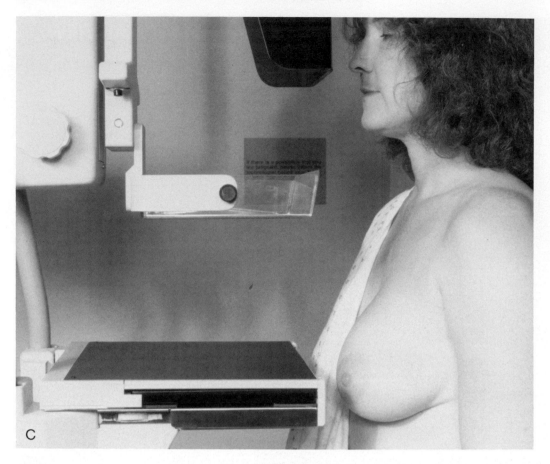

C

Figure 2-2 *Continued.* **C,** For the craniocaudal view (CC), the patient must stand facing the x-ray machine with her feet slightly apart for balance, thereby preventing motion.

D, *Top, facing page.* The technologist has greater control over the patient if she stands on the patient's side opposite the breast being positioned. In this figure, the technologist is raising the inframammary fold of the patient's left breast with her right hand. The patient's body squarely faces the x-ray machine with her face turned away from the breast being positioned. The technologist's left hand firmly guides the patient forward so that the raised IMF of the patient's breast is placed securely against the edge of the film holder. The film holder at this point should be raised to the level of the elevated IMF.

E, *Bottom, facing page.* Once the patient is firmly positioned with the IMF against the film holder, the technologist brings her left hand across the top of the left breast, and with both hands pulls the breast tissue forward from underneath and above onto the film holder. This "2-hand" technique maximizes the amount of breast tissue visualized by pulling breast tissue away from the chest wall.

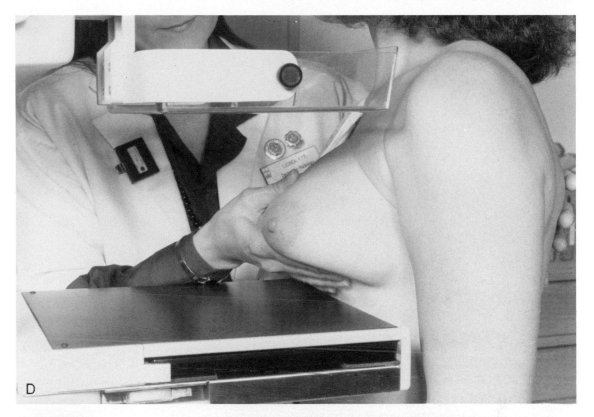

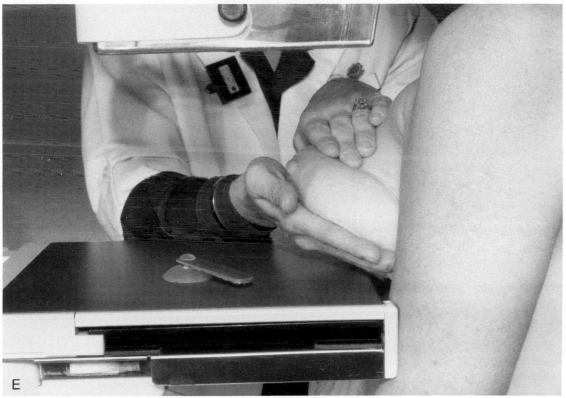

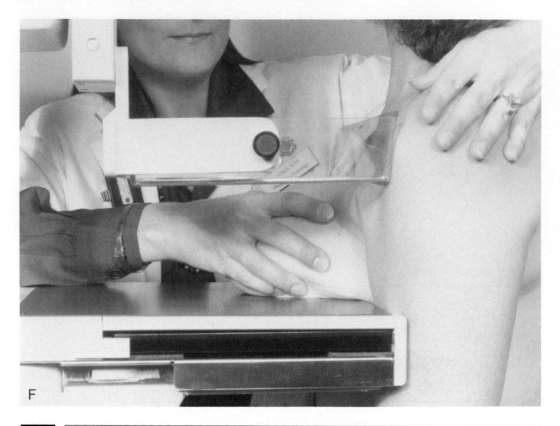

F

Figure 2-2 *Continued.* **F,** With the patient's breast firmly held on the film holder, the technologist brings her left arm around behind the patient, placing her fingers over the patient's shoulder near the clavicle. This enables the technologist to relieve any pulling sensation on the patient's skin during compression and helps the patient to keep her shoulder relaxed at the same time. As compression starts down over the breast, the technologist moves her right hand forward over the lateral breast tissue toward the nipple. This movement helps to smooth out any wrinkles, eliminate skin folds, and hold the lateral breast tissue firmly on the film holder.

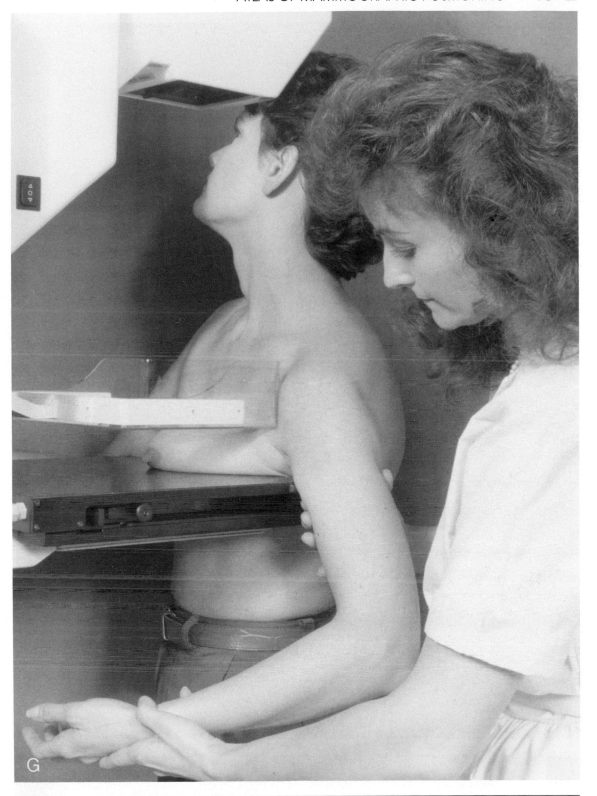

Figure 2-2 *Continued.* **G,** By externally rotating the patient's head of the humerus and having the patient's arm relaxed by her side, the technologist can also eliminate skin folds.

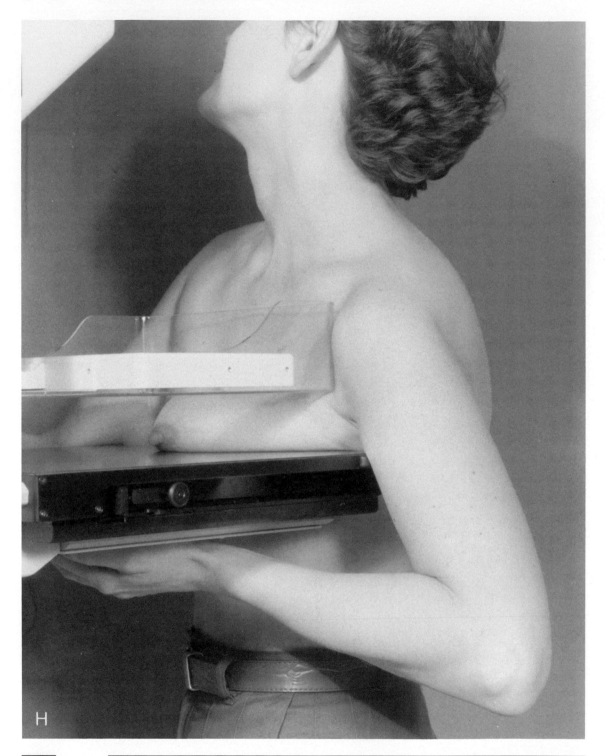

Figure 2-2 *Continued.* **H,** When working with an elderly patient who is slightly unsteady, it is acceptable to externally rotate the head of the patient's humerus and have the patient bend the elbow and gently place her hand underneath the film holder.

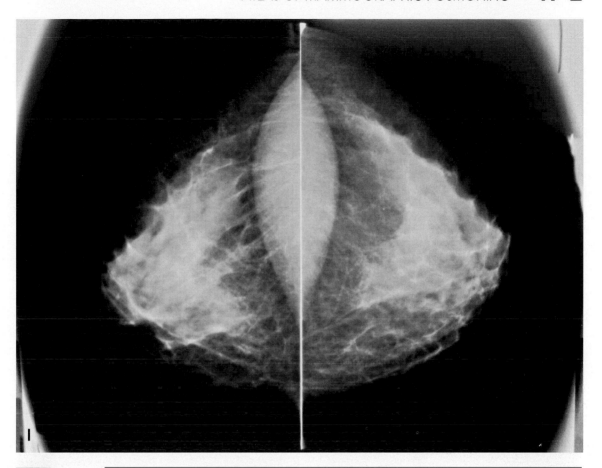

Figure 2-2 *Continued.* *I,* These radiographs are properly positioned craniocaudal views. The entire breast, including the medial, central, and much of the lateral breast tissue, is shown on the film. The patient's pectoral muscle has also been shown by adequately raising the inframammary fold. It is important to remember not to sacrifice radiographing part of the breast tissue in order to keep the nipple in profile. In some women, an additional view may be necessary to show the nipple in profile. If you have imaged more of the breast tissue with the nipple not in profile, mark "nipple not in profile" on your films. Take an additional cone-down view with the nipple in profile.

MEDIOLATERAL OBLIQUE VIEW

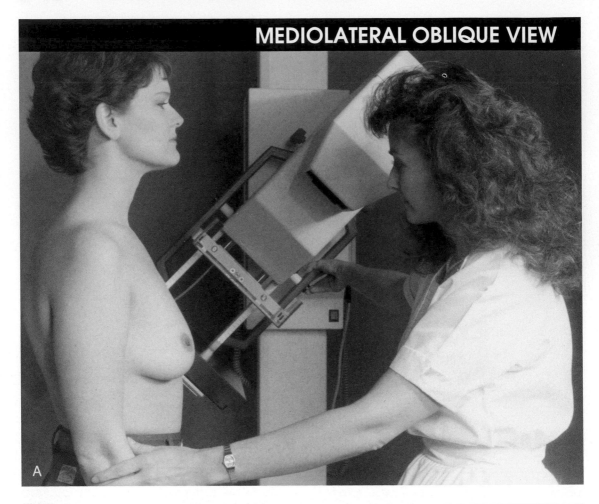

Figure 2-3. A, When the patient has been properly positioned, the mediolateral oblique view (MLO) is the single view that best images the entire breast. For this view, the technologist angles the cassette holder 30° to 60° from horizontal, making the holder parallel to the pectoral muscle. The x-ray beam is directed from the superomedial aspect to the inferolateral aspect of the breast.

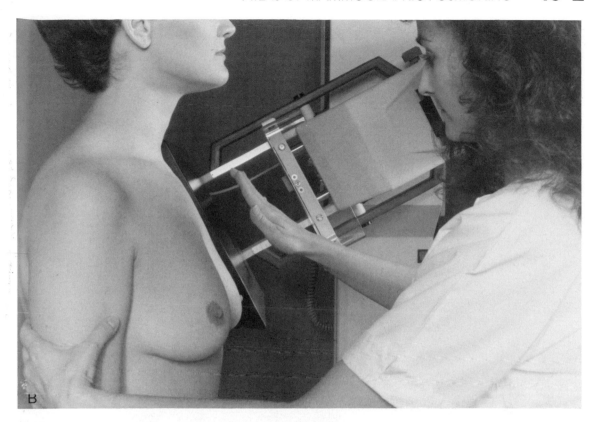

Figure 2-3. *Continued.* **B,** In this figure, the technologist is showing the angle of the patient's pectoral muscle in relationship to the film holder. Patients who are tall and thin may require a steeper angle of 55° to 60°, whereas heavy patients may require an angle of 45° to 55°. If the cassette holder is not parallel to the pectoral muscle, less breast tissue will be imaged on the film. More compression will be placed on the superior portion of the breast with less on the inferior portion of the breast. This may result in a painful examination for the patient.

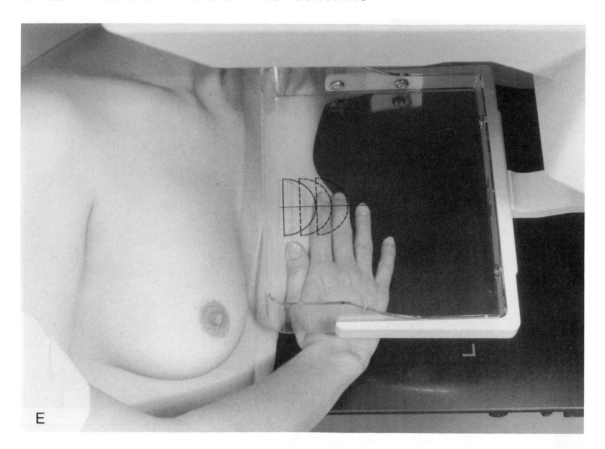

E

Figure 2-3. *Continued.* **E,** The technologist should begin applying compression while holding the patient's breast up and away from the chest wall. This technique, called the up-and-out maneuver, prevents inferior breast tissue from drooping down and being inadequately compressed because of the overlapping of breast tissue. The technologist places her arm behind the patient, with her hand resting on the patient's shoulder to ease pressure on the skin during compression. The technologist's fingers gently ease the patient's skin up over the clavicle as the compression paddle moves across the area while the technologist's arm holds the patient forward and in place.

F, Top, facing page. Full compression is shown with the superior portion of the paddle inferior to the head of the patient's humerus and the inferior portion of the paddle compressing the patient's inframammary fold. Notice how the breast is pulled straight out with no drooping on the film. If the patient has large breasts, the technologist may wish to have the patient firmly hold the opposite breast out of the way. The patient should not pull the breast or turn her body away from the machine, for this will cause breast tissue to be pulled out from the medial aspect of the breast being compressed.

G, Bottom, facing page. This figure shows a view from the back of MLO with the patient's arm resting on top of the cassette holder and her hand gently holding the handle bar. The edge of the cassette holder is placed firmly against the lateral border of the patient's breast. The patient's pectoral muscle is on the cassette holder with the latissimus dorsi just behind it.

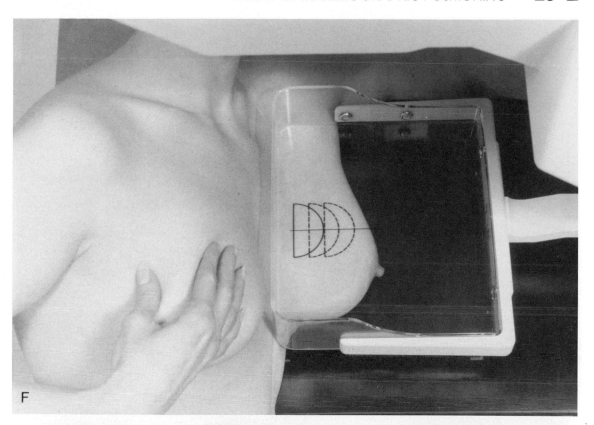

F

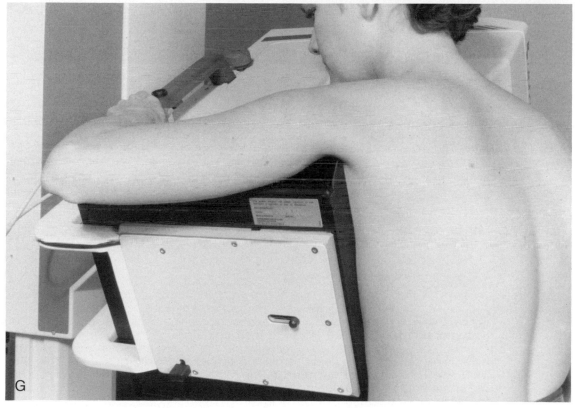

G

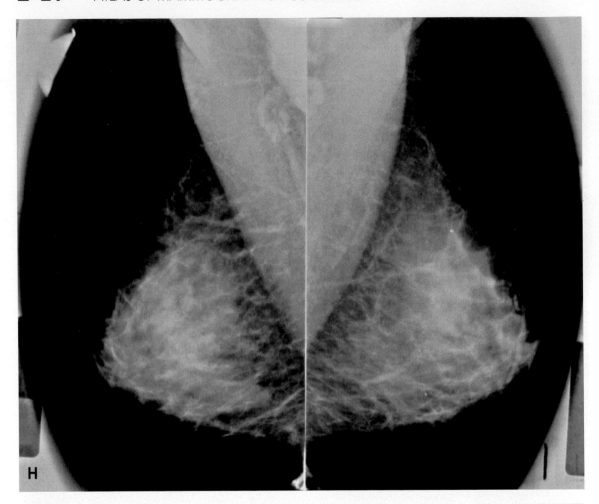

Figure 2-3.   *Continued.* ***H,*** These radiographs are properly positioned mediolateral oblique views. The pectoral muscle is seen down to the level of the nipple (1/2 to 2/3 of the way down the breast). The nipple is in profile. The breast is imaged away from the chest wall and is not drooping. Inferiorly a small portion of inframammary tissue can be seen. Remember that when the patient has been properly positioned, this view best shows the entire breast.

Figure 2-4. *A, B, Facing page.*   The posterior nipple line is the measurement on a radiograph drawn from the nipple to the back edge of the film or the pectoral muscle, whichever is first. The posterior nipple line on the craniocaudal view must be within I cm of the posterior nipple line of the mediolateral oblique, with the MLO value being the greater number. The radiographs show both the craniocaudal and mediolateral oblique posterior nipple lines as measuring 9 cm. This proves that the maximum amount of breast tissue has been imaged on both projections.

POSTERIOR NIPPLE LINE

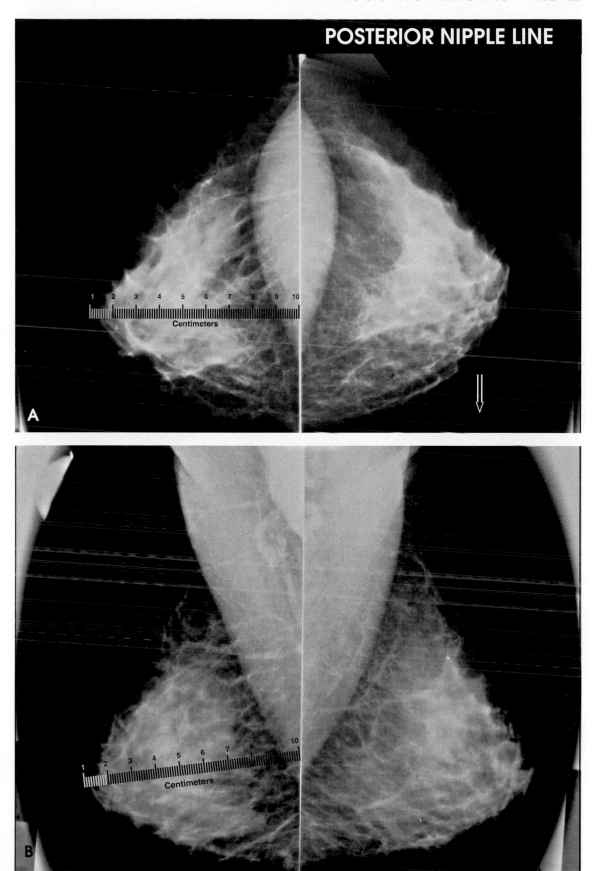

CHAPTER THREE

Modified Craniocaudal Views

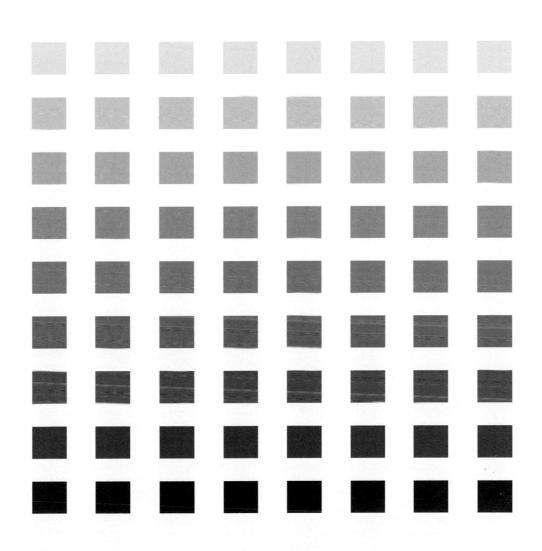

The following views will be covered in this chapter: 1) the cleavage view (CV); 2) the roll view (RM, RL); 3) the exaggerated craniocaudal view (XCCL); 4) the axillary tail view (AT); 5) caudocranial view (FB).

Figure 3-1. A, *Top, facing page.* The cleavage view (CV) may also be called the valley view. The objective of this view is to image lesions deep in the medial aspect of the breast. The technologist may position this view by standing behind the patient, reaching around to the front of the patient, and lifting both of the patient's breasts onto the cassette holder. The technologist, if standing in front of the patient, must be on the medial side of the breast being imaged. As with the regular craniocaudal view, the inframammary fold must be elevated on both breasts. Manual technique will be used if the photo sensor cell is not under a large portion of breast tissue.

B, *Bottom, facing page.* For this view, the patient's face is turned away from the breast being imaged. The technologist may want to have the patient wrap both arms along the underside of the film holder to help pull her chest wall firmly against the compression paddle and film holder. This figure illustrates a cleavage view in which the breast of interest is over the photo sensor cell so that the photo-timer may be utilized.

CLEAVAGE VIEW

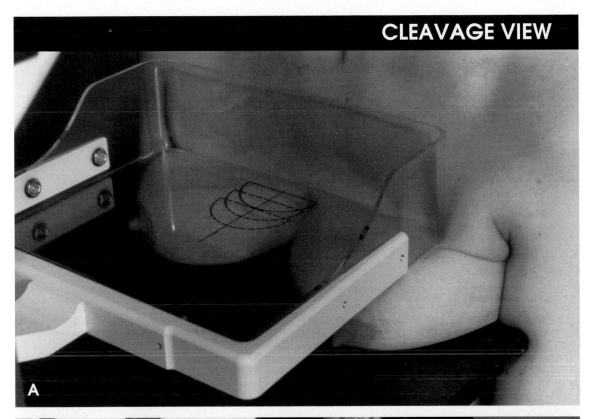

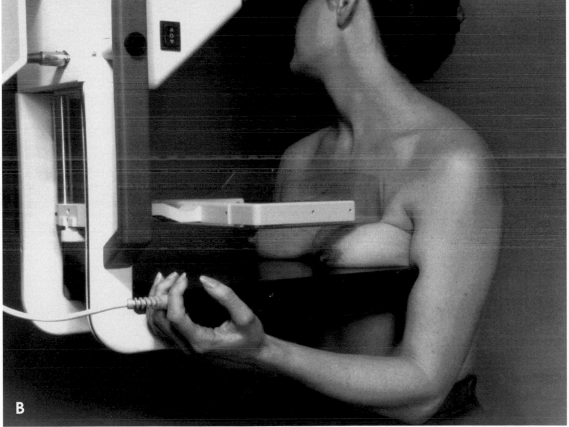

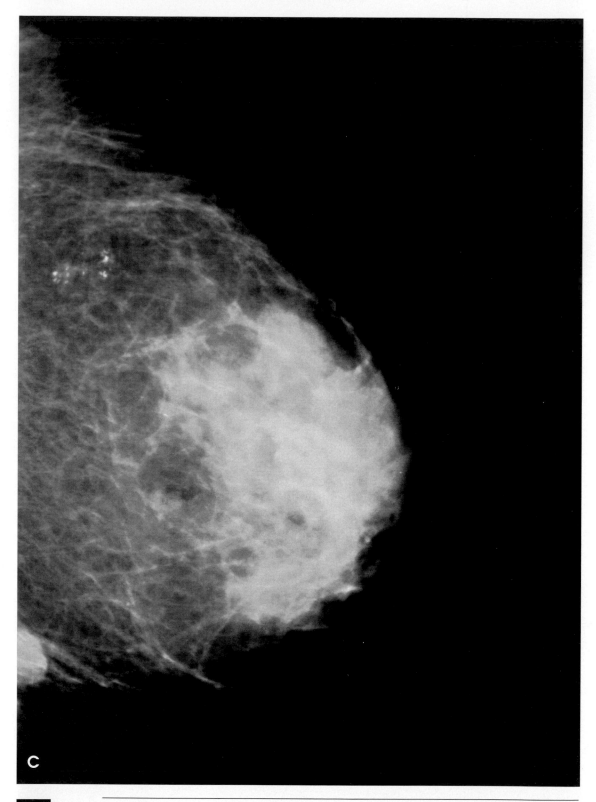

C

Figure 3-1. *Continued. C,* This radiograph is a left craniocaudal view with a partially imaged mass in the medial aspect of the breast.

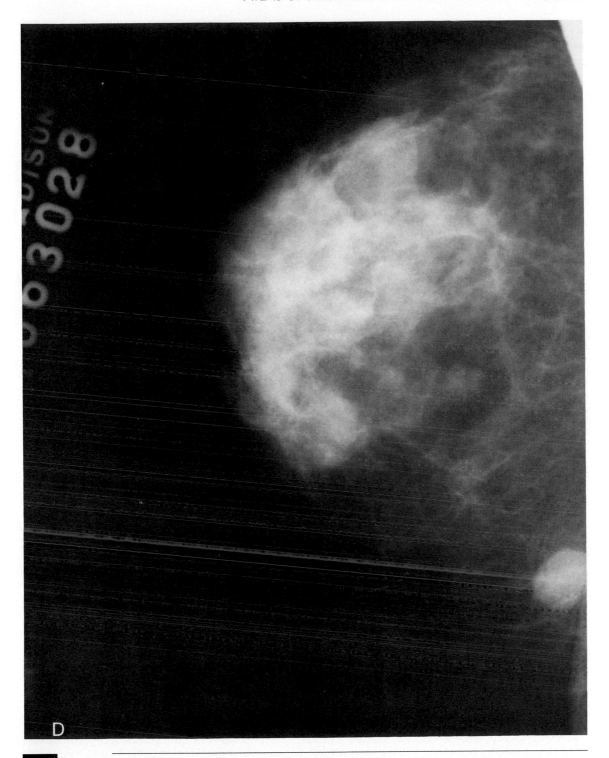

Figure 3-1. *Continued.* **D,** This radiograph is a cleavage view obtained by placing the breast of interest over the photo sensor cell with the cleavage slightly off-center. Notice that the mass in the medial portion of this breast has been better visualized than on the regular craniocaudal view. This lesion turned out to be a sebaceous cyst.

ROLL VIEW

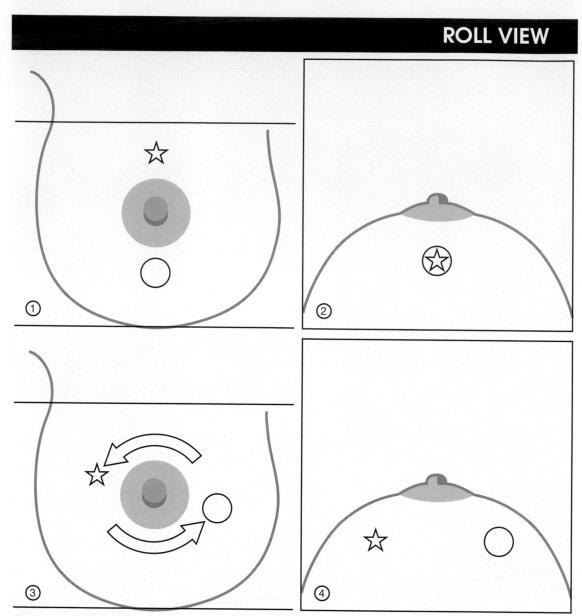

Figure 3-2. A, The roll view, either roll medially (RM) or roll laterally (RL), is utilized to separate superimposed breast tissue, confirming the presence or the absence of an abnormality on the craniocauda (CC)l view.

Illustration 1 shows the superimposition of breast tissue in the superior and inferior portion of a craniocaudal view.

Illustration 2 shows what the superimposed tissue looks like on a radiograph.

In illustration 3, the technologist places one hand on the top and the other on the bottom of the patient's breast and rolls the superior tissue laterally and the inferior tissue medially.

Illustration 4 shows what a radiograph would look like with the tissue that was superimposed having been separated, proving that the abnormality seen was not real.

B, *Top, facing page.* To perform this view, the technologist should stand on the side of the patient that the breast is to be rolled toward. The patient stands squarely facing the machine with her face turned toward the technologist as in a craniocaudal view. The technologist places one hand under the patient's breast and one hand above it, and gently lifts the inframammary fold.

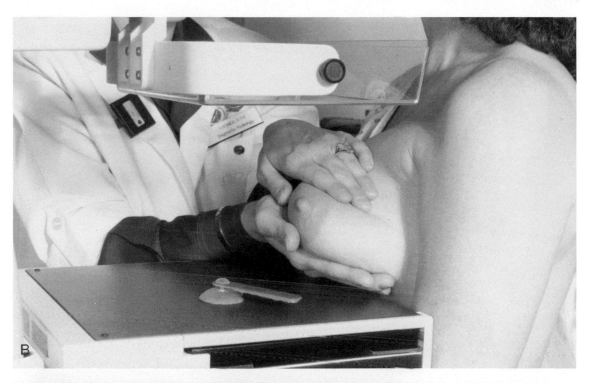

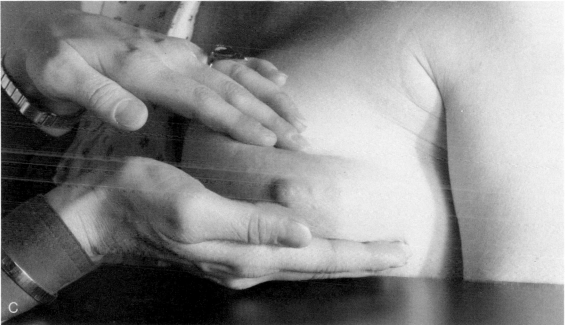

Figure 3-2. *Continued.* **C,** In this figure, the technologist is firmly rolling the patient's breast so that the superior tissue rolls medially and the inferior tissue rolls laterally. The abbreviation used on the film for this particular view is LCCRM, or left craniocaudal upper breast tissue rolled medially. Breast tissue may also be rolled in the other direction; the abbreviation for this is LCCRL, or left craniocaudal upper breast tissue rolled laterally. When a radiologist is using the roll view to better define a lesion or determine the location of a finding seen on only the CC, he or she may have the technologist perform a medial and a lateral roll view.

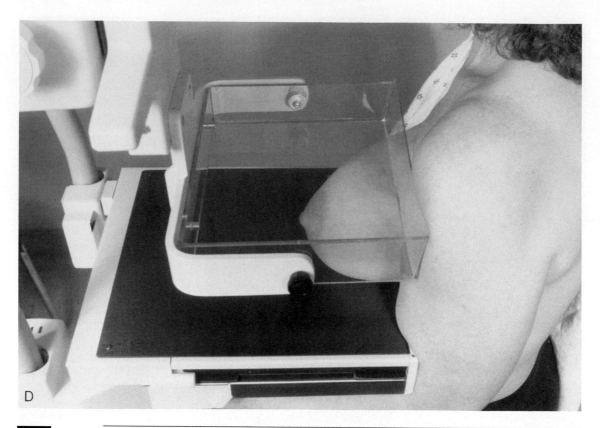

Figure 3-2. *Continued.* *D,* This figure shows a roll view with adequate compression. This view appears to be similar to a regular CC.

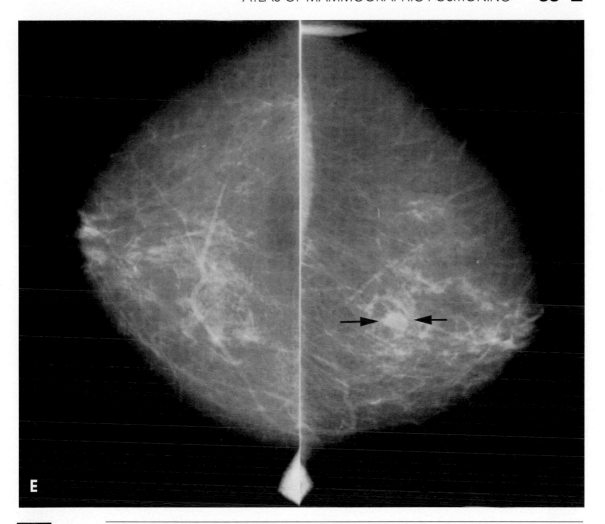

E

Figure 3-2. *Continued.* ***E,*** The radiograph on the right shows a small density in an otherwise fatty replaced breast (a nondense breast or one with little glandular tissue). The radiograph on the left shows that the technologist has used a roll view and separated the superimposed breast tissue.

EXAGGERATED CRANIOCAUDAL VIEW

A

Figure 3-3. A, The exaggerated craniocaudal view (XCCL) is used to show the outer aspect of the breast, including most of the axillary tail. Approximately 10 percent to 11 percent of all women have breast tissue that wraps around the pectoral muscle. This breast tissue may not be seen on a standard craniocaudal view. To position the patient for this view, the technologist should lift the inframammary fold and rotate the patient approximately 45° or until the lateral aspect of the breast is positioned on the cassette holder. The technologist should have the patient relax the shoulder of the breast being positioned so that it is as low as possible. The patient may hold on to the machine with the opposite arm to steady herself. A 5° lateral tube angle may be used to allow the compression paddle to clear the head of the patient's humerus. As the patient's breast is being compressed, the technologist pulls the lateral breast tissue forward onto the film with one hand while protecting the patient's clavicle with the other hand.

B, *Facing page.* This figure shows what the patient looks like during the XCCL.

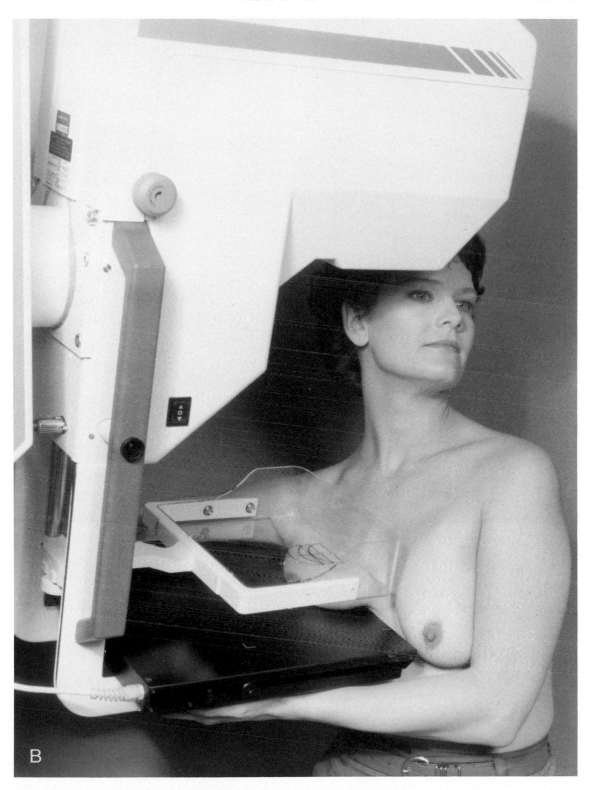

B

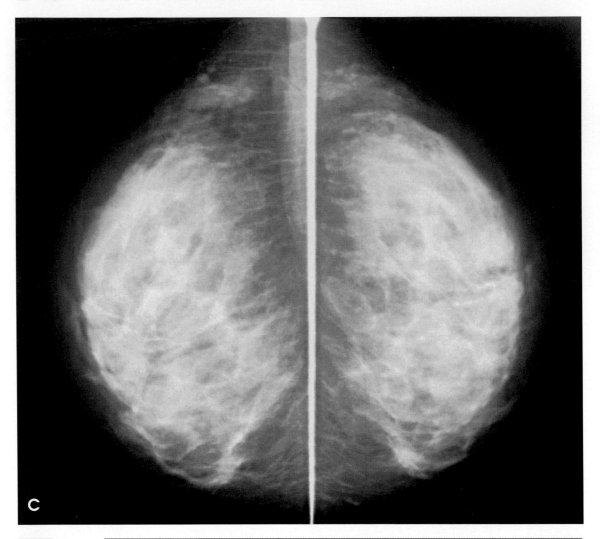

C

■

Figure 3-3. *Continued.* **C,** The radiograph on the right is a standard left cranio-caudal view (CC). Breast tissue is seen going off the film in the lateral aspect of the breast. The radiograph on the left is the same breast positioned with a 5° lateral tube angle utilizing the XCCL. A small amount of pectoral muscle has been imaged as well as the island of glandular tissue located in the upper outer quadrant of the left breast.

■

Figure 3-4. A, *Facing page.* The axillary tail view (AT), previously called the cleopatra view, demonstrates the entire axillary tail and lateral aspect of the breast. This view will not show the inframammary fold of the breast, although it looks similar to a medio-lateral oblique view on the radiograph. The tube and cassette holder are angled to parallel the pectoral muscle at an angle between 30° and 50°. The patient's arm rests along the top of the film holder with the shoulder completely relaxed. The technologist lowers the height of the C-arm until the superior edge of the compression paddle is just below the head of the patient's humerus. The technologist spreads the axillary portion of the patient's breast up and out with her hand as compression is applied. It is important that the patient have her pectoral muscle relaxed while this maneuver is being done. This ensures that the deep structures of the axilla will move forward away from the chest wall and onto the cassette holder. The patient's opposite arm may remain at her side or the patient may bend the arm at the elbow, bracing the hand under the cassette holder for better balance.

AXILLARY TAIL VIEW

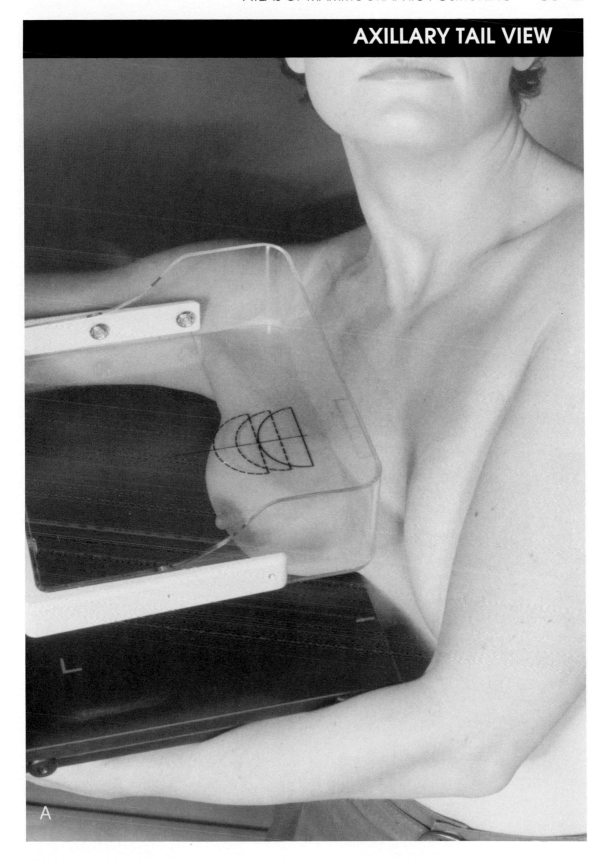

A

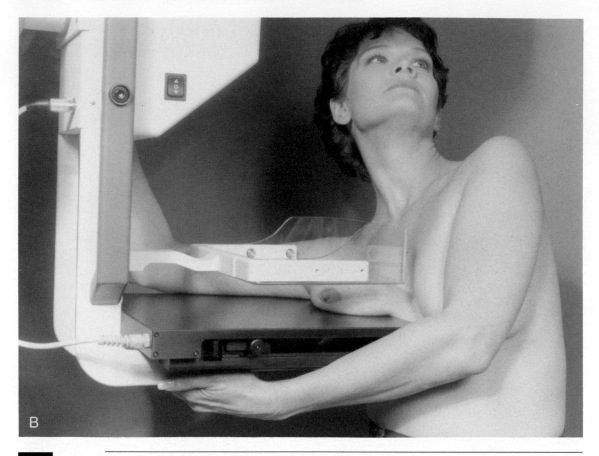

B

Figure 3-4. *Continued. B,* This figure depicts the way the patient used to be positioned for the cleopatra view. This was difficult for even the most agile patient. In experimenting with this position, it was discovered that if the tube arm was rotated while the patient slowly stood up, the technologist could adequately visualize the axillary tail with far less discomfort to the patient.

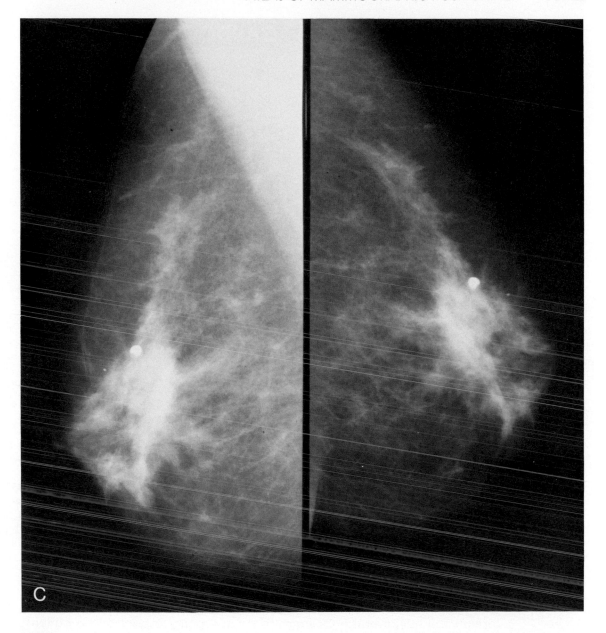

Figure 3-4. *Continued.* **C,** The radiograph on the right is a properly positioned craniocaudal view. The radiograph on the left is the same breast with a 30° lateral tube angle utilizing the axillary tail view. This projection appears to be similar to a mediolateral oblique; however, as stated before, no inframammary fold has been imaged.

CAUDOCRANIAL VIEW

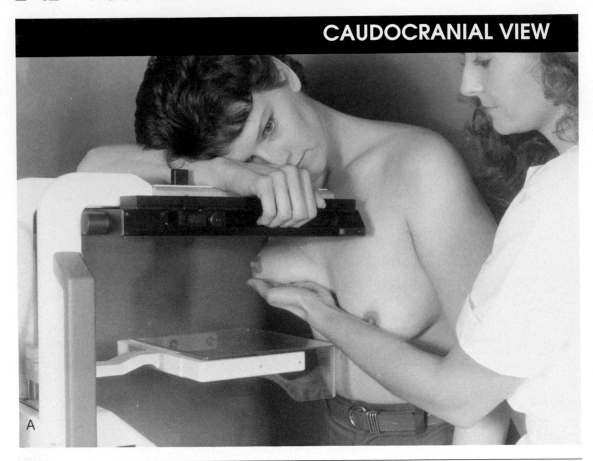

A

Figure 3-5. *A,* This figure shows a caudocranial view (FB), a reverse craniocaudal view in which the tube is rotated 180° and the x-ray beam is directed from below: thus the abbreviation *FB.* This view is excellent for women with small breasts and patients with severe kyphosis. It may also be used for preoperative needle localization for lesions located in the most inferior portion of the breast, or as a contact view for lesions located in the superior aspect of the breast. For this view, the patient stands facing the unit with her legs on either side of the tube head. The patient bends slightly forward from the waist while resting her face and arm on the bottom of the film holder. This ensures that no abdomen is imaged in the field of view. The technologist raises the inframammary fold and adjusts the height of the C-arm so that the superior aspect of the patient's breast is firmly on the cassette holder. As compression is applied, the technologist will move her hand slowly toward the patient's nipple, spreading the breast forward onto the cassette holder.

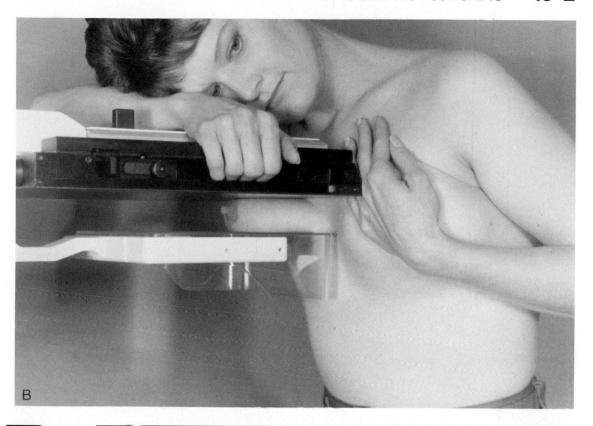

B

Figure 3-5. *Continued.* **B,** This figure shows a caudocranial view (FB) with adequate compression applied to the breast. Notice that the medial portion of the breast that is *not* being imaged is hanging slightly over the edge of the compression paddle, ensuring the imaging of all of the medial tissue of the breast being compressed. If the patient has large breasts, the technologist may want to have her gently hold the opposite breast out of the field of view.

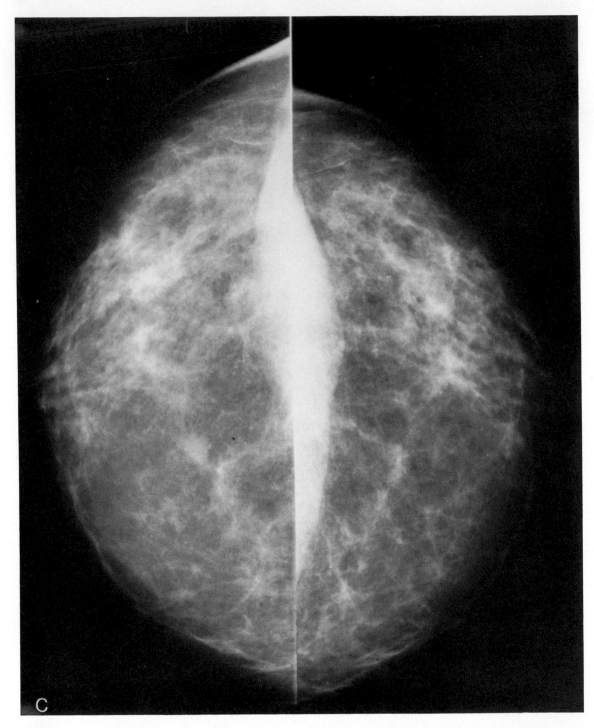

C

Figure 3-5. *Continued.* ***C,*** These radiographs are properly positioned right and left caudocranial views on a kyphotic patient. Notice the large amount of pectoral muscle imaged on each film.

CHAPTER FOUR

Modified Lateral
Views

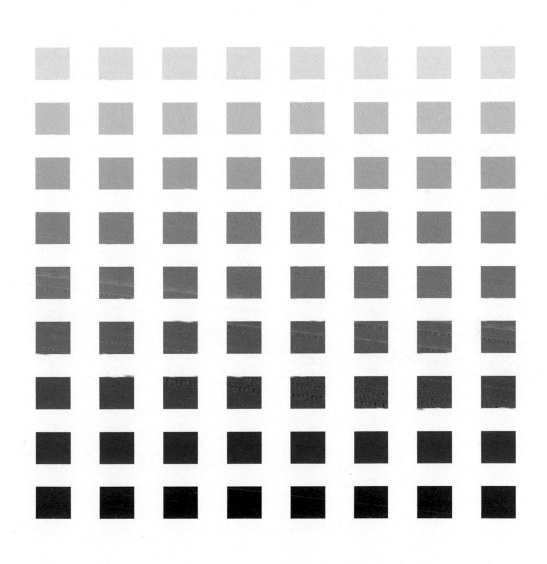

This chapter covers 1) the 90° mediolateral view (ML); 2) the 90° lateromedial view (LM); 3) the lateromedial oblique view (LMO); 4) the superolateral to inferomedial oblique view (SIO); and 5) the tangential view (TAN).

THE 90° LATERAL VIEW

The most commonly used additional view is the 90° lateral view, whether mediolateral or lateromedial. The 90° lateral view helps the radiologist to triangulate the exact location of a lesion previously seen only on the mediolateral oblique view of a screening study. If a lesion moves down relative to the nipple on a 90° film or is lower than it was on the oblique film, the lesion is in the lateral aspect of the breast. However, if the lesion moves up relative to the nipple or is higher than it was on the mediolateral oblique film, the lesion is in the medial aspect of the breast. If the location of the lesion has not significantly changed on a 90° film, the lesion is located in the central portion of the breast.

True lateral films, either medial or lateral, also reduce geometric unsharpness by placing the lesion closest to the film. For example, a lesion seen in the medial aspect of the breast on a craniocaudal view would best be demonstrated by utilizing the 90° LM.

90° MEDIOLATERAL VIEW

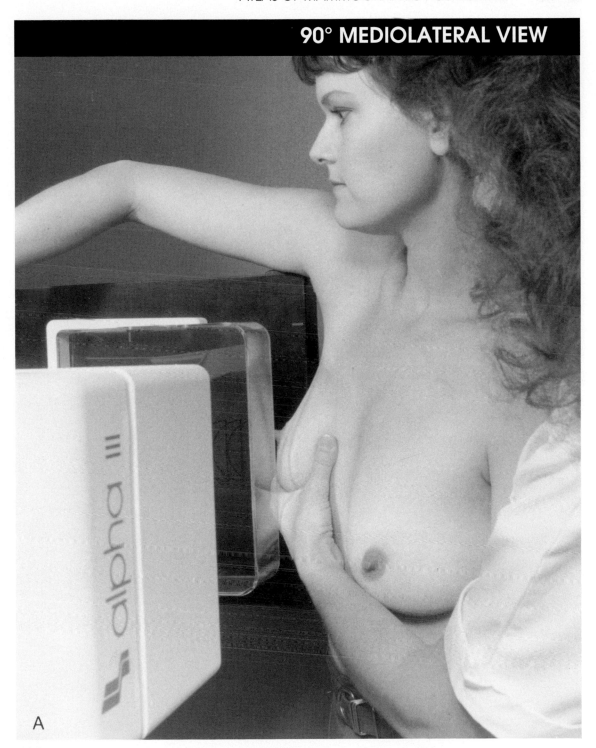

A

Figure 4-1. A, The technologist begins the mediolateral view (ML) by rotating the tube head to a true 90° angle. The patient faces the machine, reaching across the cassette holder to gently hold the handlebar. At the same time, the technologist stands at the patient's opposite side and guides the hollow of the axilla onto the corner of the cassette holder.

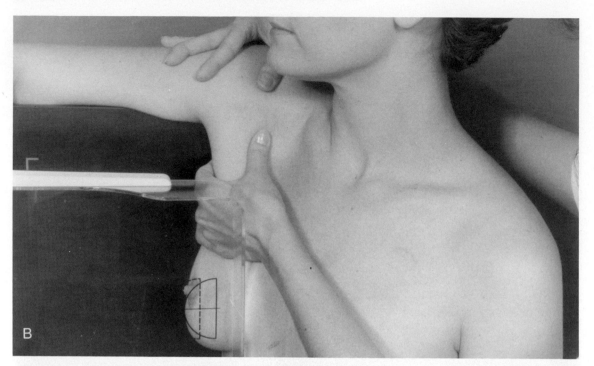

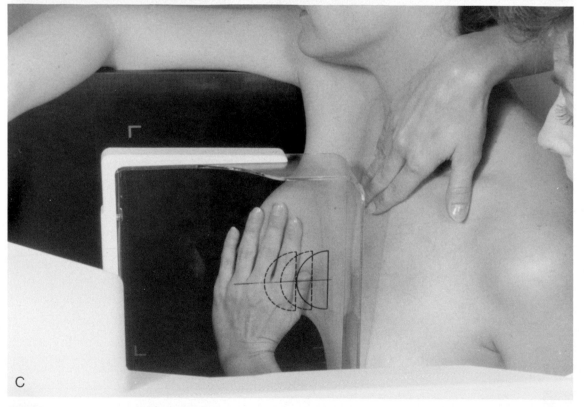

Figure 4-1 *Continued.* ***B,*** *Top.* Once the patient's underarm is in contact with the edge of the cassette holder, the technologist should make sure the patient's pectoral muscle is relaxed with the shoulder resting firmly on top of the cassette holder. If the patient's pectoral muscle is tense, adequate compression of the entire breast will be difficult and the patient may experience quite a bit of discomfort.

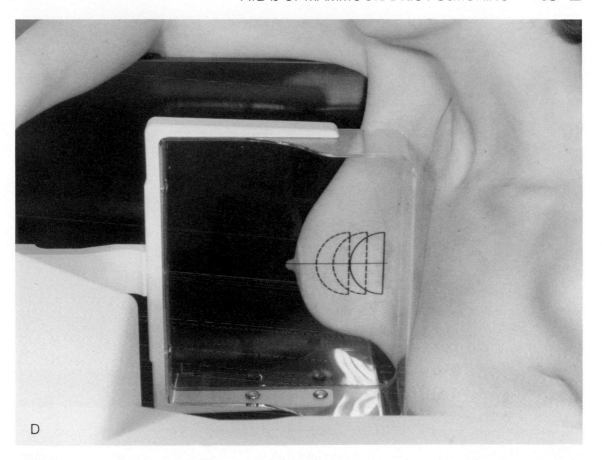

D

Figure 4-1 *Continued. C, Bottom, facing page.* As with the mediolateral oblique view (MLO), the technologist should utilize the principle of the mobile versus fixed margin of the breast by lifting the patient's breast tissue and pectoral muscle medially toward the sternum. The technologist should then rotate the patient down onto the cassette holder until the breast is firmly held in place. The technologist should use the up-and-out maneuver to hold the breast in place as compression is engaged, being careful to gently ease a little skin out as the paddle slides down over the sternum.

D, Above. This figure shows how the 90° mediolateral position looks prior to the x-ray exposure. The nipple is in profile, with the breast being pulled up and out from the chest wall. The inframammary fold has been opened by gently pulling abdominal tissue down. The anterior edge of the compression paddle is firmly against the sternum.

If the patient has large breasts, she may be required to gently hold the opposite breast out of the way during exposure. The technologist must make sure that the patient does not pull the breast or rotate her shoulder out, which would pull breast tissue out from under the edge of the compression paddle.

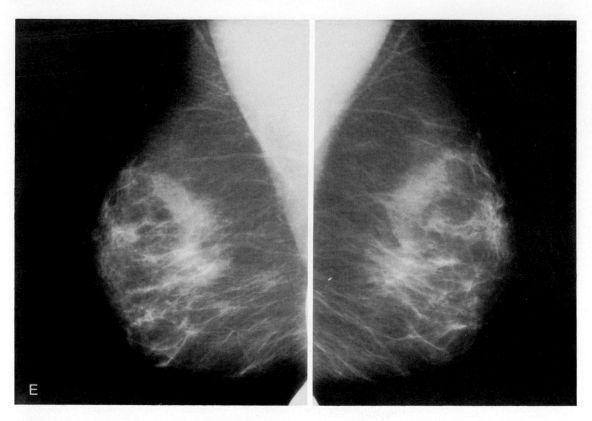

E

Figure 4-1 *Continued.* ***E,*** The radiograph on the left is a properly positioned 45° MLO. The pectoral muscle has been imaged down to the level of the nipple. The breast has been pulled up and out, and there is excellent compression separating all structures. The radiograph on the right is a 90° ML. Less pectoral muscle has been imaged and the glandular tissue is shown in a slightly different projection and is more compressed because there is not as much pectoral muscle pulled forward onto the film.

90° LATEROMEDIAL VIEW

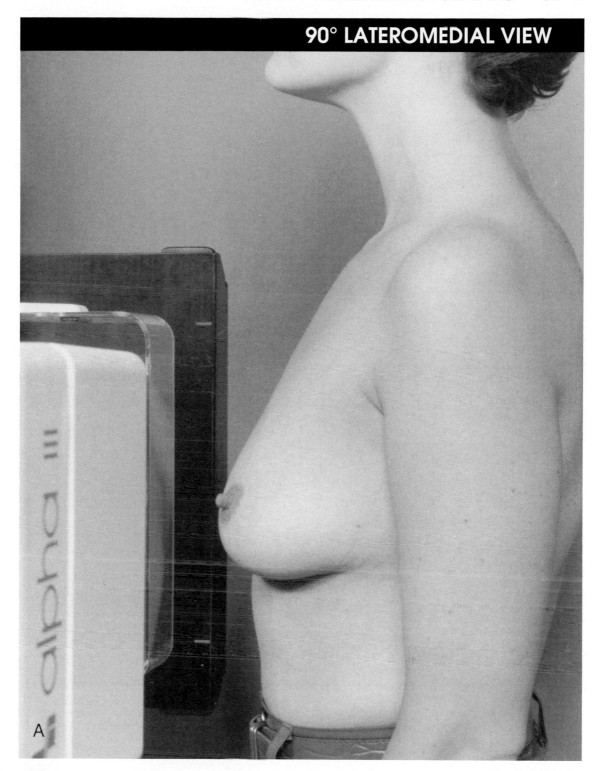

Figure 4-2. A, To position a patient for a 90° lateromedial view (LM), the technologist rotates the tube head to 90°. The patient faces the machine while the technologist raises the film holder until the edge is at the level of the suprasternal notch.

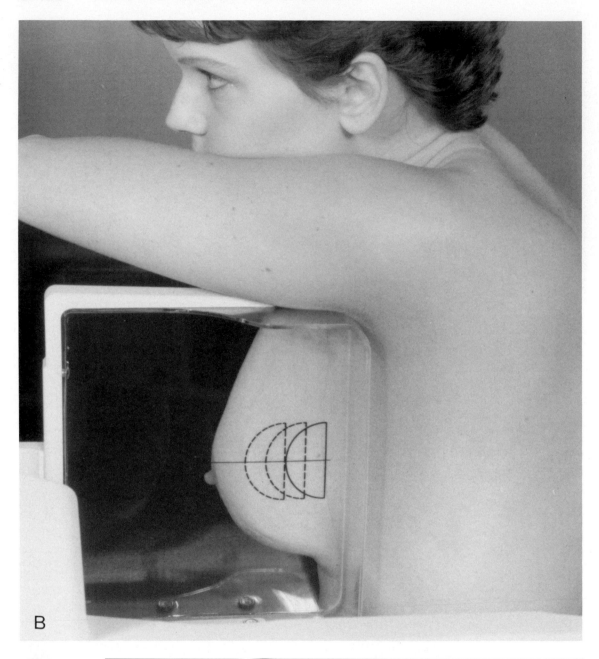

B

Figure 4-2 *Continued.* **B,** In this figure, the patient is positioned so that her sternum is in contact with the cassette holder. Her neck is extended forward with her chin resting on the edge of the cassette holder. The arm on the side of the breast being positioned should rest over the cassette holder with the elbow flexed to relax the pectoral muscle. The patient is rotated slightly medially as the technologist pulls the breast up and out onto the cassette holder while the compression paddle begins its descent. The edge of the compression paddle passes in front of the latissimus dorsi muscle and rests firmly on the pectoral muscle. If the patient has a large skin flap on the underarm, it may be necessary for her to raise the arm as the technologist compresses the breast to avoid catching the skin of the arm under the compression paddle. The technologist must always remember to open the inframammary fold by smoothing the abdominal tissue down.

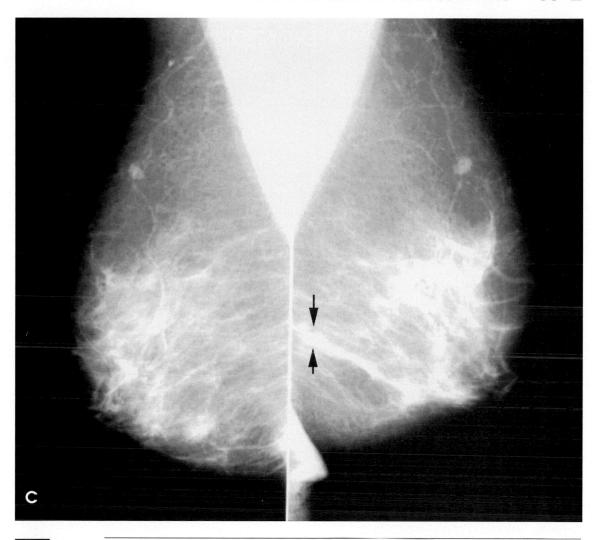

Figure 4-2 *Continued.* **C,** The radiograph on the left is a 60° mediolateral oblique view (MLO). This image was taken on a patient with pectus excavatum; the patient's breast bone is concave, making imaging of medial breast tissue extremely difficult. Notice that a fair amount of pectoral muscle, but absolutely no inframammary fold, has been imaged. The radiograph on the right is a properly positioned 90° LM on the same patient. The pectoral muscle is seen to the same extent as that on the MLO, but on this radiograph the inframammary fold, as well as more medial breast tissue, has been imaged. Notice the small density (indicated by arrows) seen on this view that was not visualized on the MLO.

LATEROMEDIAL OBLIQUE VIEW

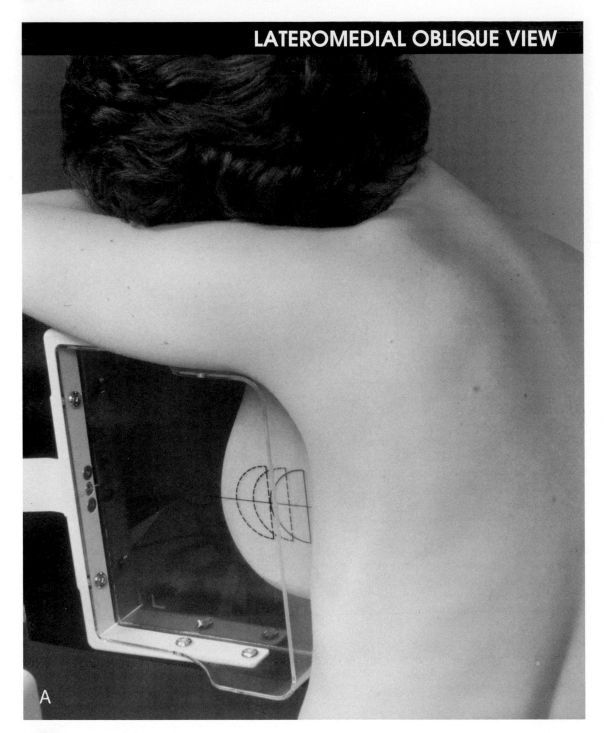

Figure 4-3. *A,* This figure shows a properly positioned lateromedial oblique view (LMO). It is a true reverse oblique because the x-ray beam is directed from an inferolateral to a superomedial direction. The cassette holder and compression paddle are parallel to the pectoral muscle as with the mediolateral oblique (MLO), thus ensuring the imaging of a large amount of breast tissue. This view is positioned in a fashion similar to the 90° lateromedial view and is also a contact view.

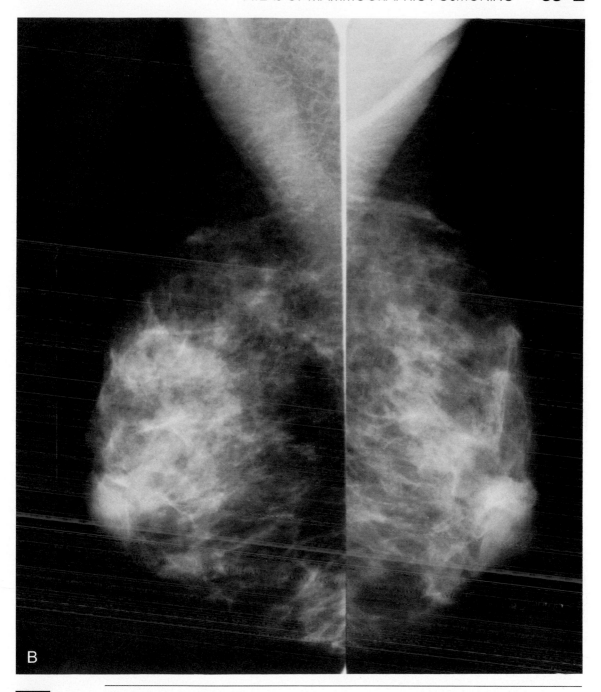

B

Figure 4-3 *Continued.* **B,** The radiograph on the right is a 50° MLO on a patient with severe pectus excavatum. It is obvious that there is an inadequate amount of breast tissue imaged on this radiograph. The radiograph shows only a small amount of pectoral muscle with no inframammary fold, and medial breast tissue is cut off by the posterior edge of the film. The radiograph on the left is a properly positioned 50° LMO on the same patient. The pectoral muscle has been adequately imaged and the inframammary fold is seen. The medial breast tissue that was cut off by the edge of the film in the other projection is now seen in the central aspect of the breast. The LMO may also be used for patients who have had recent open heart surgery or who have a prominent pacemaker. This view may also be beneficial for patients with a kyphotic curvature of the spine.

SUPEROLATERAL TO INFEROMEDIAL OBLIQUE VIEW

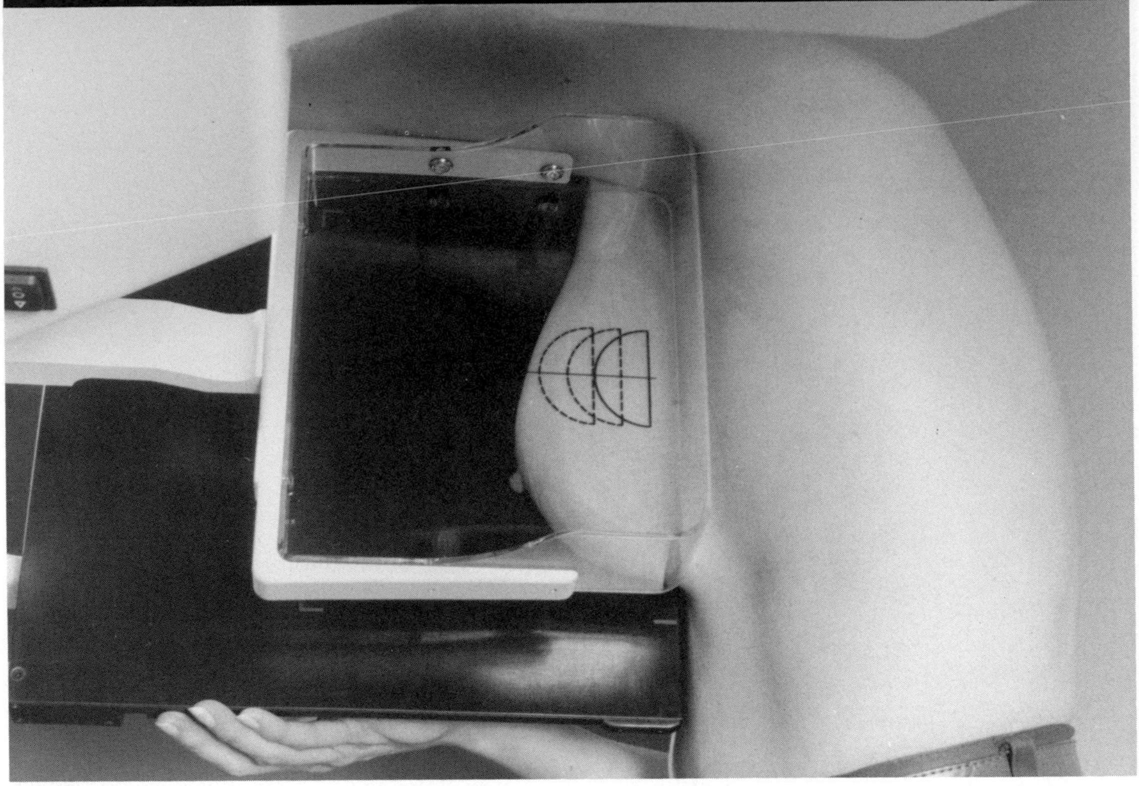

Figure 4-4. This positioning is for the superolateral to inferomedial oblique view (SIO), which for years was incorrectly termed the reverse oblique view. It is positioned with the x-ray machine's central ray directed from the superolateral to the inferomedial aspect of the breast. The cassette holder and compression paddle work against the angle of the pectoral muscle. Normally, very little inframammary fold is imaged. This view has limited usefulness and is included here as an example of what *not* to do.

Figure 4-5. *A, Facing page.* If the patient presents with a palpable lesion that is obscured by dense glandular tissue on the mammogram, a tangential view (TAN) may be of use to the radiologist. To obtain this view, the technologist places a lead marker directly over the lump. The C-arm is then rotated until the x-ray beam is tangential to the lead marker. This maneuver places the palpable lump away from the glandular tissue and into the subcutaneous area of the breast with the lead marker being seen at the skin line. The technologist must hold the patient's breast firmly in place as compression is engaged, thus keeping the lead marker on the skin line.

TANGENTIAL VIEW

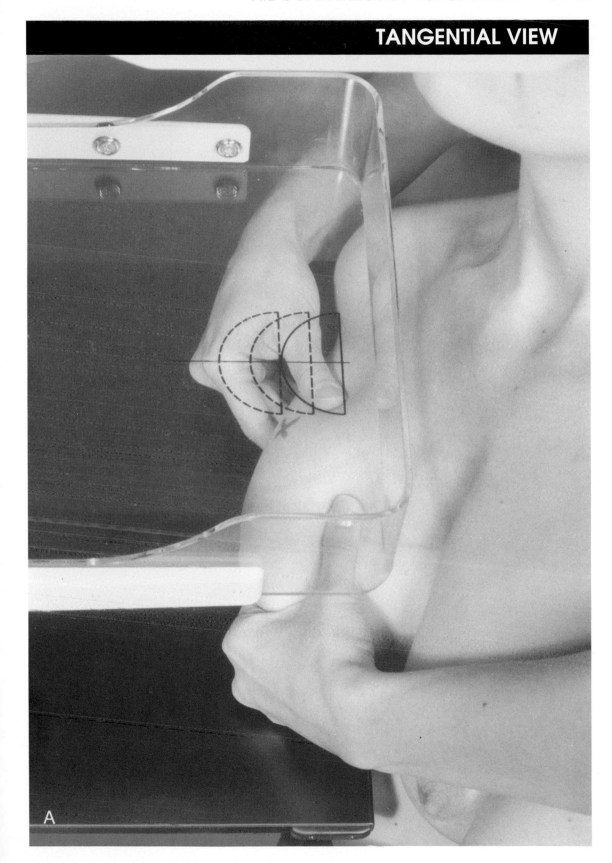

A

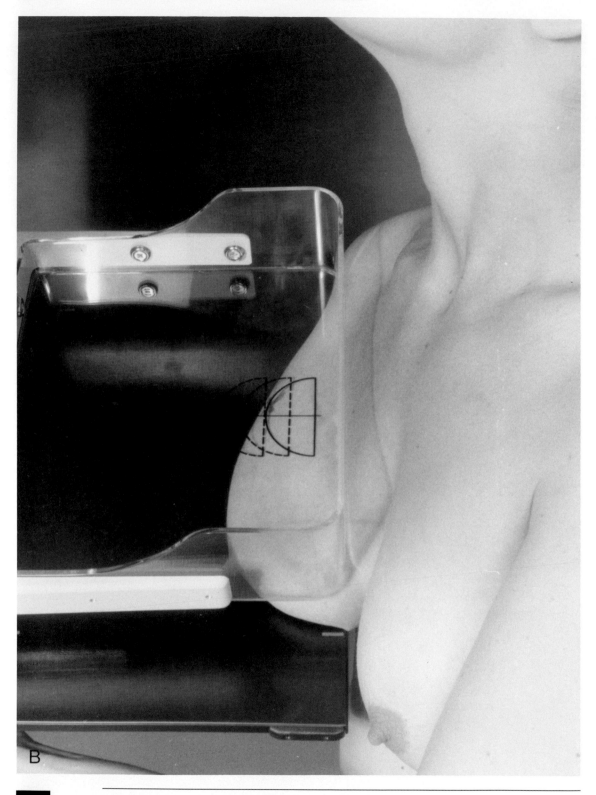

Figure 4-5 *Continued. **B,*** Some radiologists may want the technologist to include the nipple on this view for orientation purposes. Full breast compression is then needed.

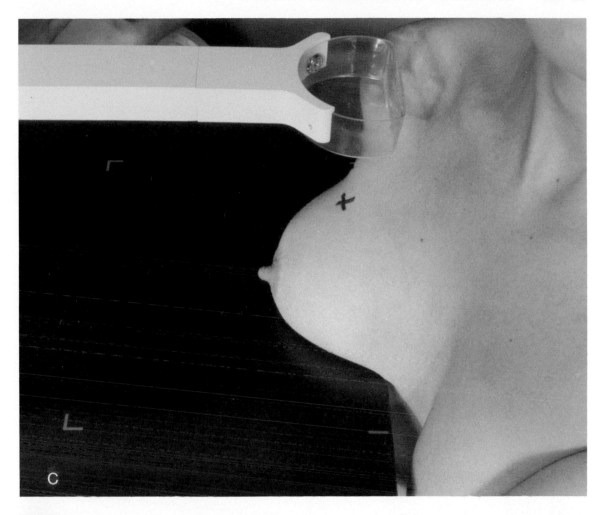

Figure 4-5 *Continued.* **C,** Spot compression is often used with the tangential view. This enables better compression of the area in question and reduces geometric unsharpness.

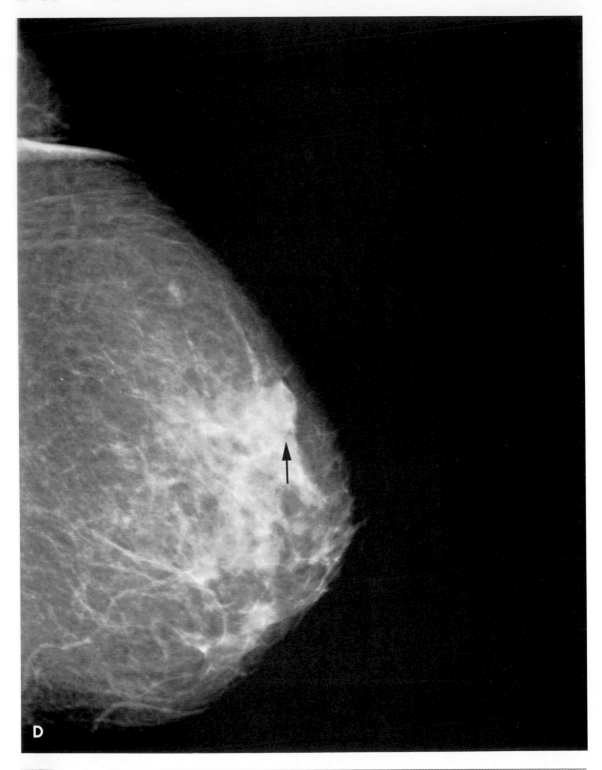

Figure 4-5 *Continued.* ***D,*** This radiograph is a craniocaudal view (CC) of a patient with a palpable breast lump. The arrow indicates an area of increased density that must be studied further.

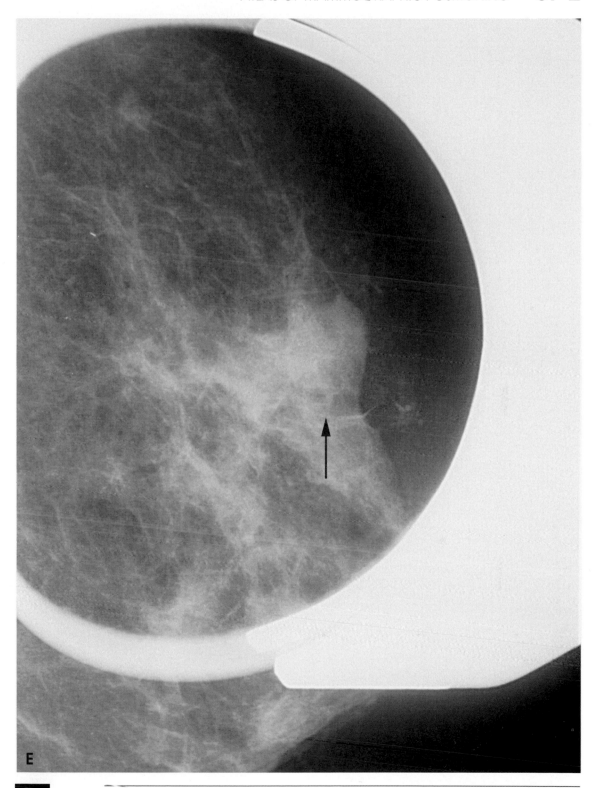

E

Figure 4-5 *Continued.* *E,* This is a radiograph of a tangential view utilizing spot compression. The breast lump is over more of the subcutaneous fat, allowing better visualization. This (arrow) lesion has irregular borders and was sent for biopsy. The findings were positive for cancer.

CHAPTER FIVE

A Special Technique for Microcalcifications and Small Masses

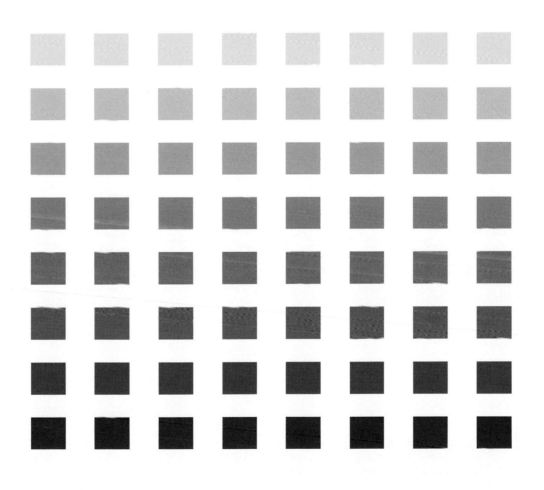

This chapter discusses the use of spot compression with and without magnification. The benefits of magnification are also covered.

■

Figure 5-1. *A, Facing page.* This is a radiograph of a craniocaudal view (CC) that shows a suspicious density with irregular margins (arrows). A spot or cone compression view would be an ideal complement to this study. Spot compression reduces thickness of breast tissue and separates structures in a localized area of interest. Using the original craniocaudal view, the technologist must use the nipple as a landmark for locating the area to be compressed. I find the finger technique to work well.

SPOT COMPRESSION VIEWS WITHOUT MAGNIFICATION

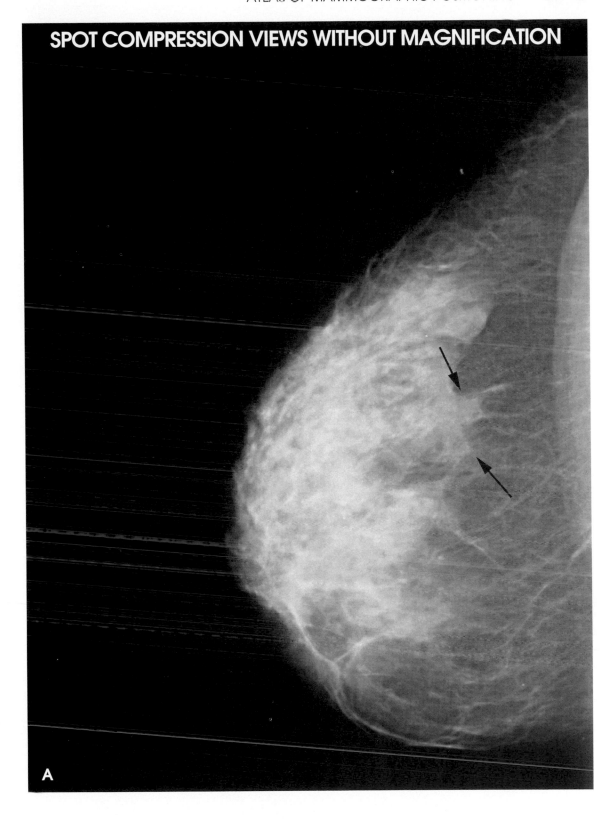

A

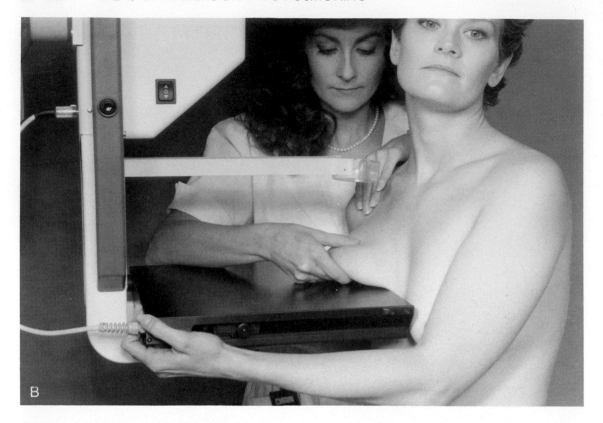

B

■

Figure 5-1 *Continued.* **B,** For this view, the technologist places the patient's breast on the cassette holder, using the same techniques as for the original craniocaudal view. If the patient held onto the machine with one hand, she should do so again. If her chin was up or down, the position should be copied exactly. Small changes in the original position may cause the technologist to miss part of the area of interest under the spot compression.

    C, *Top, facing page.* Using the nipple for a reference, the technologist measures how far laterally she has to compress the breast to image the area of interest. In this figure, the technologist is holding two fingers to the lateral portion of the breast.

    D, *Bottom, facing page.* From that point the technologist must find out how far back from the nipple to the chest wall she has to compress the breast.

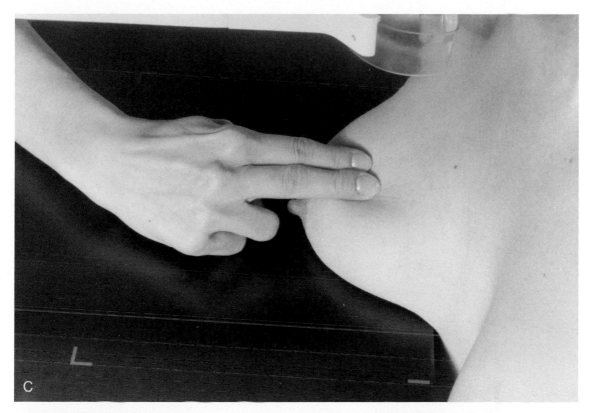

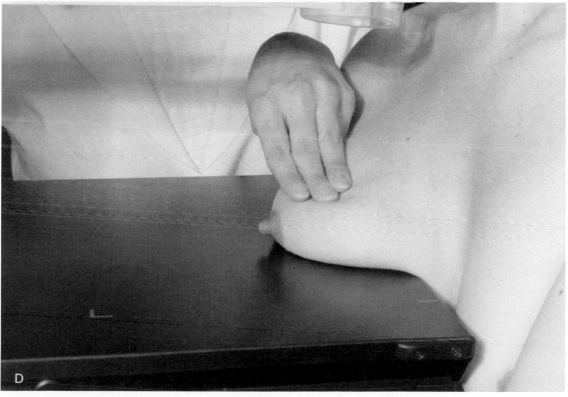

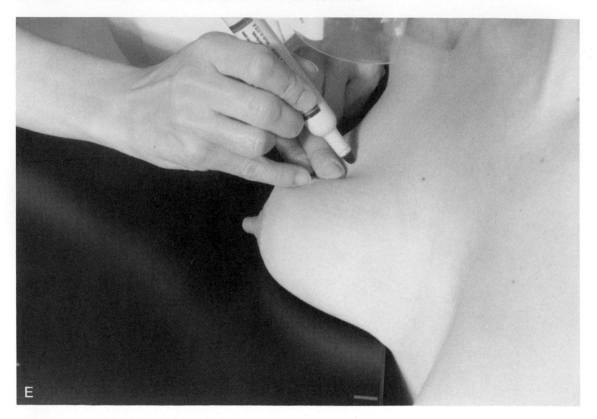

E

Figure 5-1 *Continued.* ***E,*** A felt-tip pen is used to mark the location of the area of interest on the breast surface. The technologist should center the compression paddle directly over this area.

F, *Top, facing page.* The technologist must firmly hold the breast onto the film holder as compression is engaged, making sure that the area of interest is directly under the center of the spot compression device.

G, *Bottom, facing page.* This is a radiograph of spot compression in a cranio-caudal view. Laterally the arrow shows a small ovoid density. This density was proven to be a fibroadenoma on biopsy. Medially the arrows show a density with irregular borders. This density was proven to be a carcinoma on biopsy.

This irregular, asymmetric tissue was biopsied and proved to be normal glandular tissue.

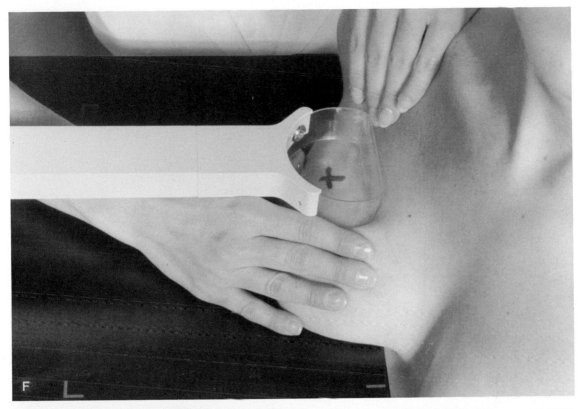

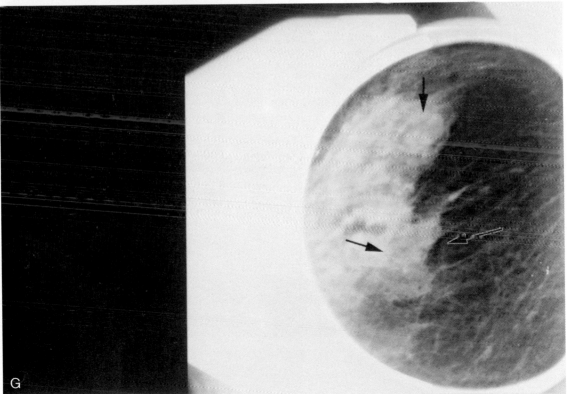

SPOT COMPRESSION VIEW WITH MAGNIFICATION

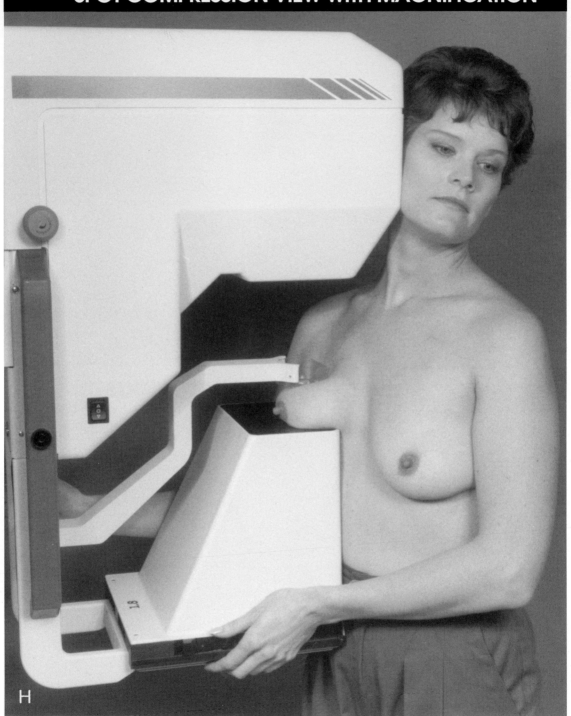

Figure 5-1. *H, Facing page.* Spot compression may also be utilized with magnification. Magnification enables the radiologist to evaluate the margins and other architectural characteristics of a focal mass. It also permits better delineation of number, distribution, and shape of calcifications. Magnification requires an x ray tube with a measured focal spot size of no more than 0.2 mm (0.1 mm is preferred), because an increase in object-to-film distance causes geometric unsharpness. The greater the level of magnification, the smaller the focal spot required. In this figure, the patient is positioned on a magnification platform or tower. The grid has been removed because the air gap resulting from the separation of the breast from the image receptor reduces the amount of scattered radiation. In magnification mammography, long exposure times are used. It is critical that the patient remain still for the duration of the exposure. Patients who have trouble holding their breath may not be suitable for magnification views.

CHAPTER SIX

Visualizing the Breast Tissue of a Mastectomy Patient

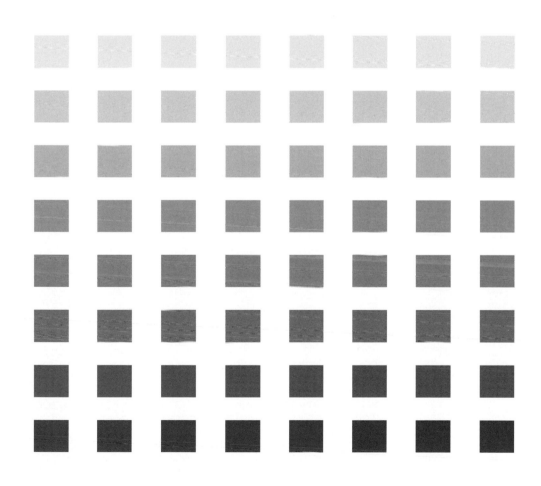

The two views discussed in this section are the retromammary view and the postmastectomy axillary view. Both of these views are used to check for recurrence of cancer in the axilla and along the chest wall incision.

Figure 6-1. **A,** *Top, facing page.* To position the patient for the postmastectomy axillary (skin flap) view, the technologist adjusts the C-arm on the machine to an angle that matches the pectoral muscle. The technologist places the patient in the mediolateral projection with the patient's elbow bent and her arm extended across the film holder at a 90^0 angle. The technologist stands at the patient's opposite side and guides the hollow of the axilla onto the cassette holder the same as is done for the mediolateral oblique view. The technologist places the corner of the cassette holder behind the patient's pectoral muscle with the patient's latissimus dorsi muscle behind the film holder. The technologist then rotates the patient forward onto the film holder and activates compression.

B, *Bottom, facing page.* This figure shows what the finished position looks like. Notice that the superior edge of the compression paddle is located posteriorly to the head of the patient's humerus and that the sternum is pressed firmly against the posterior edge of the compression paddle. The phototimer may be used if enough breast tissue covers the sensor cell, but the technologist may need to set a manual technique.

SKIN FLAP VIEW

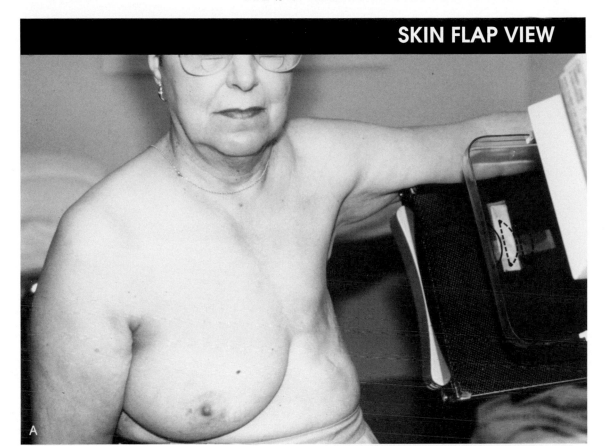

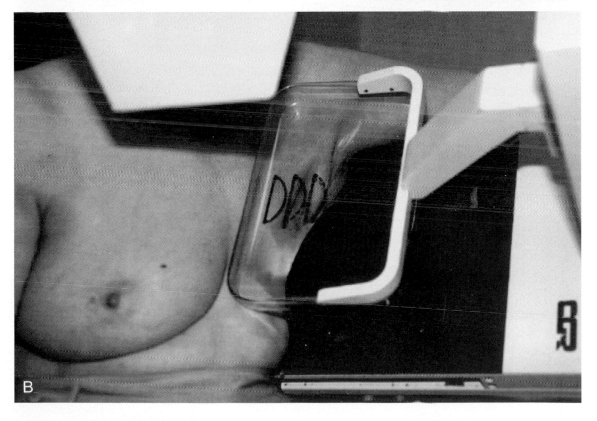

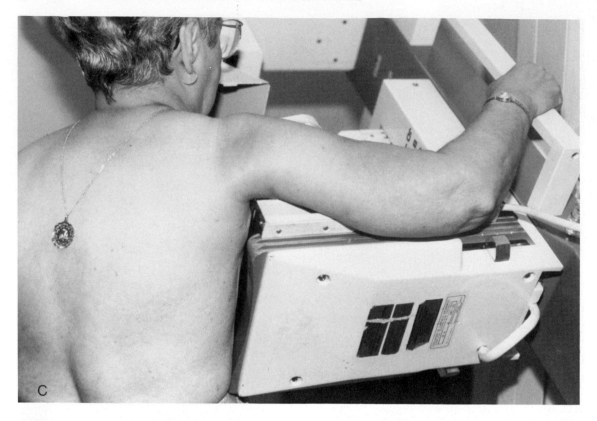

Figure 6-1. *Continued. C, Above,* This figure shows the view from behind the patient. The patient's arm is relaxed on top of the cassette holder, and the corner of the film is securely in the axilla.

D, Facing page. This radiograph shows the pectoral muscle and surgical incision of a postmastectomy patient.

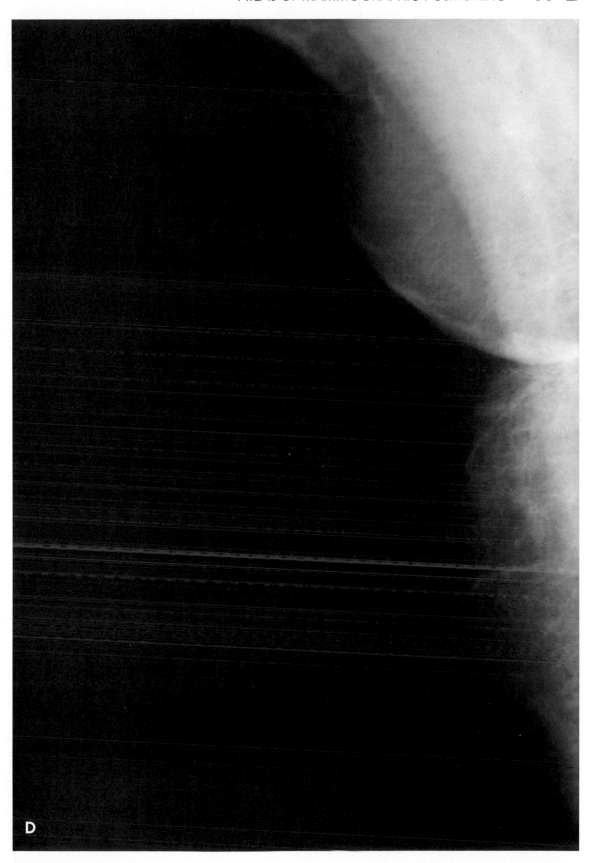

D

RETROMAMMARY VIEW

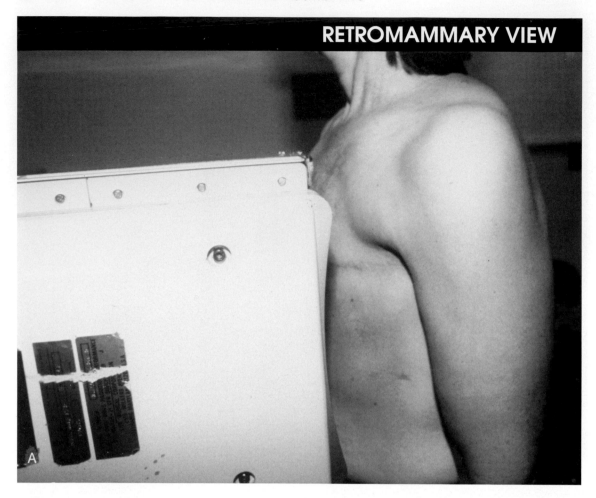

Figure 6-2. *A,* The retromammary view images bone detail in the rib and humeral areas as well as the retromammary space and subcutaneous tissue. For this position, the technologist rotates the machine to a 90° true lateral position.

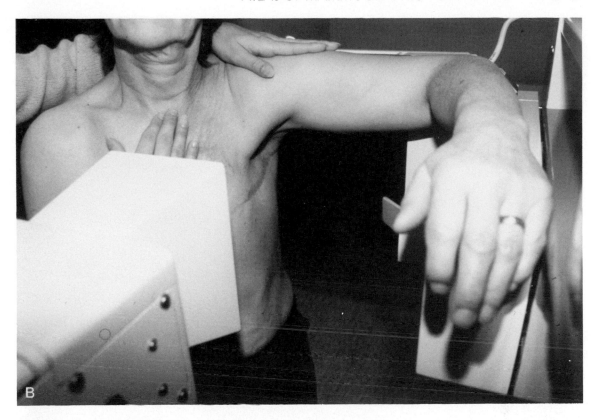

Figure 6-2. *Continued. **B,*** The technologist places the patient in an anteroposteri-or position on the film holder. The patient's arm is abducted in a 90° angle from the body with the elbow bent and the forearm resting on the handlebar. Because the compression paddle is removed for this view, the technologist will find ample space for placing the patient in this position. The technologist then raises the C-arm until the top of the film holder is at the top of the patient's humerus.

C, *Page 80.* This is a properly positioned retromammary view on a mastecto-my patient. Notice the soft tissue detail from the head of the humerus down along the rib cage. This view is also helpful when imaging the posterior edge of an implant, because it is not seen on a routine exam. This view can be obtained best with mammography machines that have aluminum filters. The aluminum filter gives the technologist the correct kilovoltage setting for penetrating the bony structures.

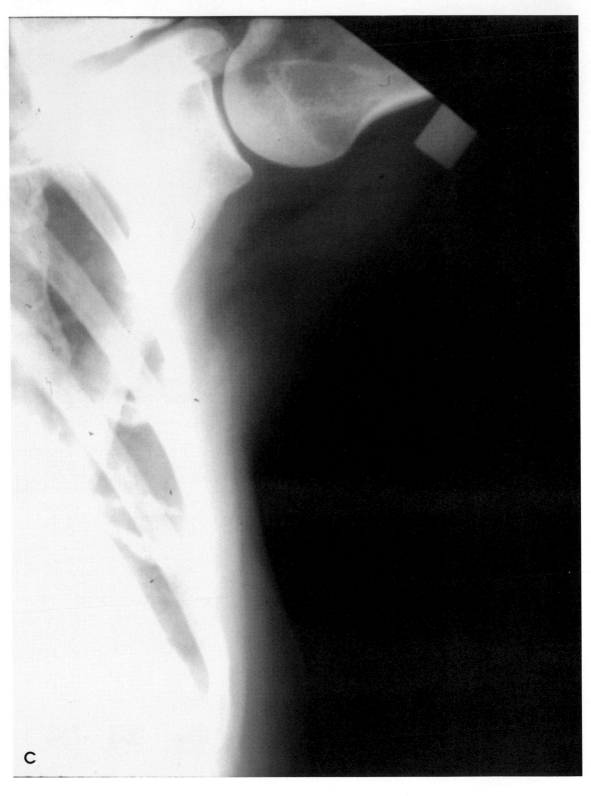

C

CHAPTER SEVEN

Tips for Difficult-to-Position Patients

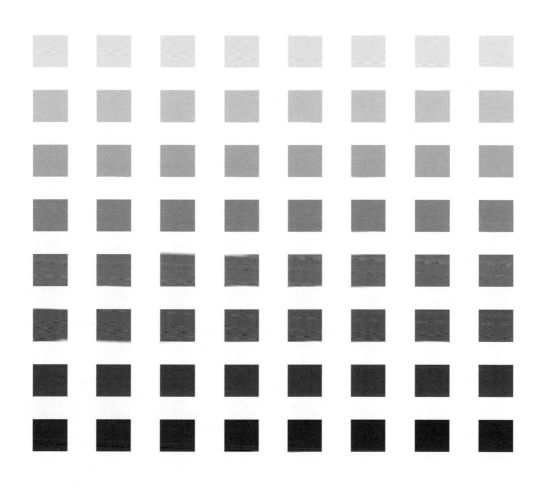

This chapter covers
1. cart patients
2. wheelchair patients
3. male mammography
4. imaging the augmented breast.

Creativity and imagination are useful when dealing with special circumstances in the mammography suite.

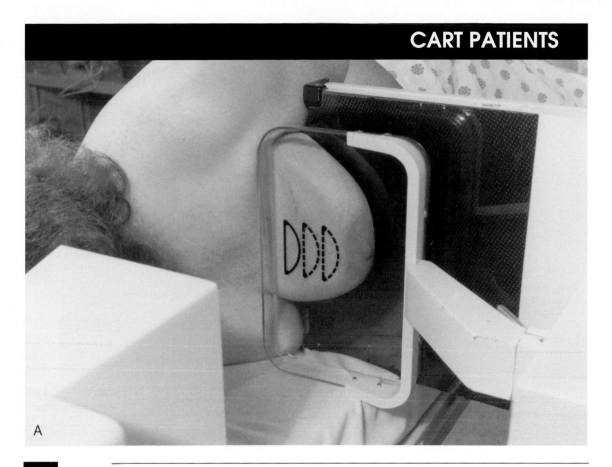

CART PATIENTS

A

Figure 7-1. A, When a patient is unable to stand or sit upright for mammography, excellent films may be obtained by using the x-ray machine's ability to rotate to any angle necessary. In this figure, the patient is positioned for a craniocaudal view (CC) on the left breast. The patient lies on her right side with her right arm up under her head, which is placed on a pillow. The patient's legs are bent at a 45° angle for balance. The machine's C-arm has been rotated to 90°. The technologist is most successful standing behind the film holder and reaching across to hold the patient's breast on the film holder. The patient's inframammary fold has been elevated slightly, as with a regular craniocaudal view. Lateral breast tissue is well compressed and the patient's left arm is relaxed at her side, with the elbow bent so that the palm of her hand may be turned up resting on the underside of the cassette holder. Notice that the opposite breast has not been pulled firmly back but left to rest slightly over the edge of the film holder; thus, this view images more medial breast tissue on the breast of interest.

Figure 7-1 *Continued.* **B,** *Facing page.* A 90° lateromedial view (LM) has been obtained as the complementary view to the craniocaudal view. In this case, the machine's C-arm remains at 0°. To obtain this position, the patient remains turned on her right side, with her head resting on a pillow. Both of her arms are abducted at a 90° angle from the body, with the elbows bent and the forearms resting on the cart. The left breast has been lifted laterally with the film holder between the breasts in the cleavage area. The patient is rolled slightly forward onto the film holder, and compression is obtained with the posterior edge of the compression paddle sliding along the lateral border of the patient's rib cage. Notice that the inframammary fold, as well as much of the pectoral muscle, has also been placed onto the film holder. Whether the patient has an injured back or must remain recumbent for other reasons, the technologist is able to image a large amount of breast tissue by keeping the patient stable and relaxed. Sometimes placing a pillow between the patient's knees helps the patient feel more balanced. The technologist must remember to keep the side rail on the cart up behind the patient for safety. The brakes on the cart should also be locked before the compression paddle has been fully engaged.

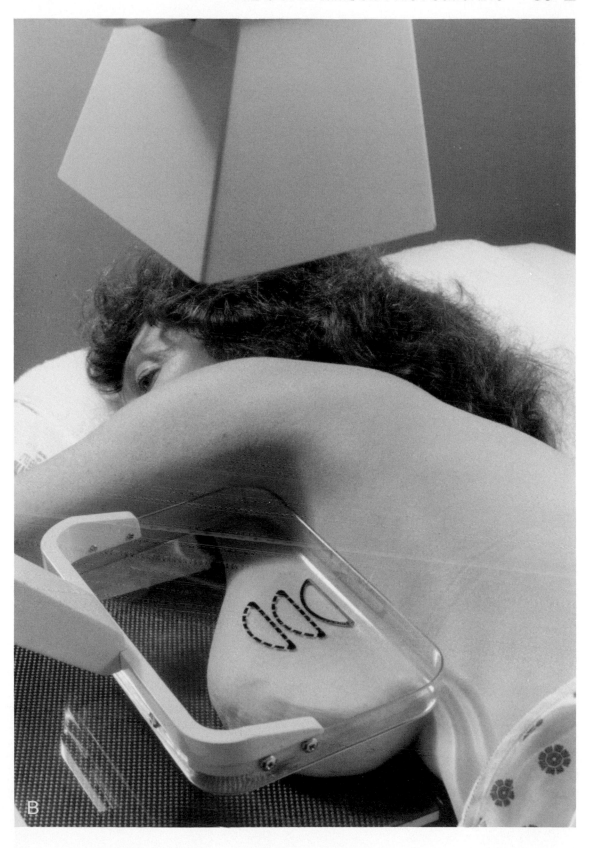

B

WHEELCHAIR PATIENTS

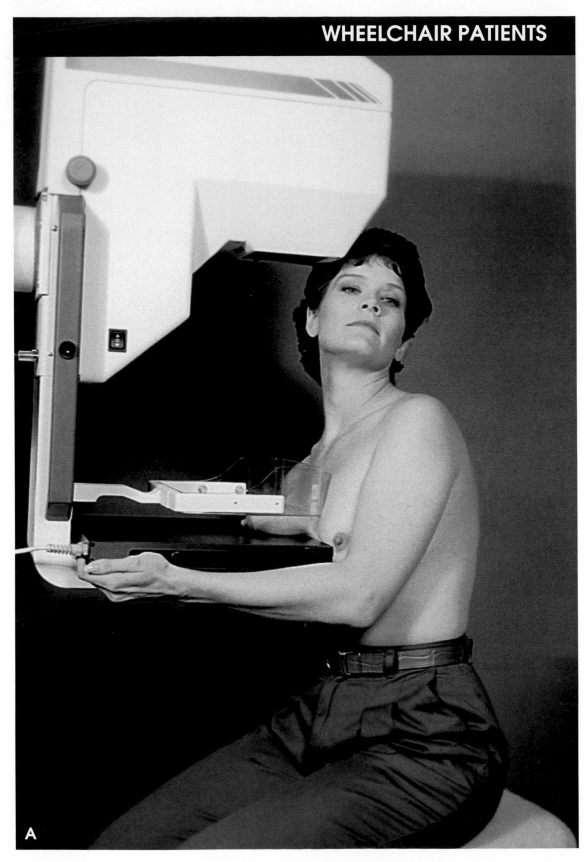

A

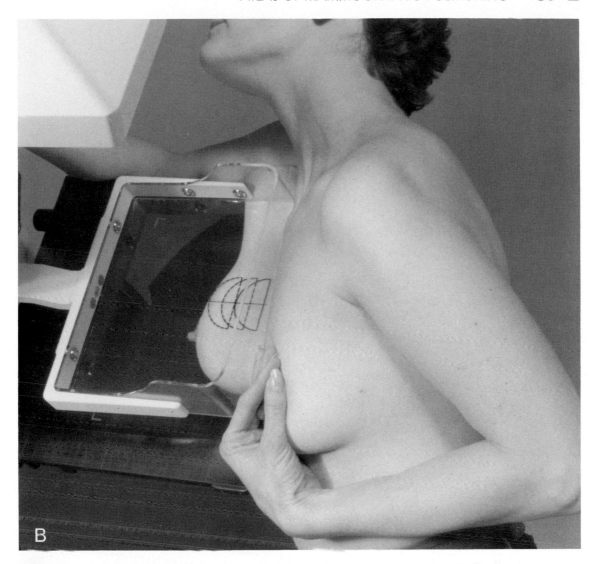

Figure 7-2. A, *Facing page.* Patients who are in wheelchairs pose a different problem. This figure shows the patient positioned for the craniocaudal view (CC) while seated. It is helpful to the technologist if the patient is able to wrap her arms around the underside of the cassette holder and grasp its edges. Leaning the patient forward will enable the technologist to pull the patient's breast away from the chest wall and onto the cassette holder. It may be necessary for the technologist to prop the patient's back up with sponges or pillows, thereby leaning the patient slightly forward in the wheelchair for easier access to her breast. The technologist should always lock the wheelchair brakes before leaving the patient alone in this position.

B, *Above,* A mediolateral oblique view (MLO) or lateromedial oblique view (LMO) may be used as a complement to the CC for a wheelchair patient. Once again it is important to have the patient leaning forward while seated. The breast is easier to position on the film holder if it is slightly pendulous and away from the chest wall and abdomen. It may be wise to use two technologists when working with a patient in a wheelchair or on a cart. This enables one technologist to steady the patient and position the breast while the other technologist sets the technique to be used on the control panel and engages the compression paddle.

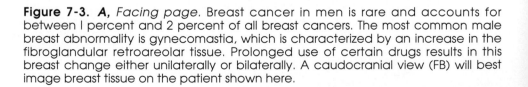

Figure 7-3. A, *Facing page.* Breast cancer in men is rare and accounts for between I percent and 2 percent of all breast cancers. The most common male breast abnormality is gynecomastia, which is characterized by an increase in the fibroglandular retroareolar tissue. Prolonged use of certain drugs results in this breast change either unilaterally or bilaterally. A caudocranial view (FB) will best image breast tissue on the patient shown here.

MALE MAMMOGRAPHY

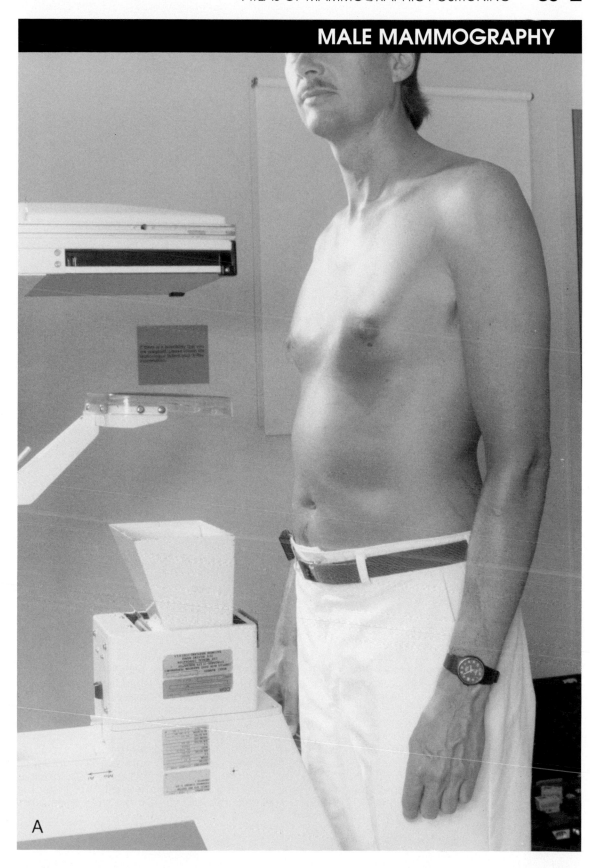

A

Figure 7-3 *Continued.* ***B,*** *Facing page.* To perform this procedure, the technologist must rotate the C-arm 180°. The patient faces the unit with one leg on each side of the tube head. The patient's inframammary fold should be elevated and the height of the machine's C-arm adjusted so that the superior border of the breast is in contact with the cassette holder. The patient should extend his neck forward and rest his chin on the bottom of the film holder. The patient's arm should also be abducted away from the body and draped over the bottom of the cassette holder in a relaxed position. Using the palm of the hand or a spatula, the technologist spreads the patient's breast up and out onto the film holder as the compression paddle is engaged. (A rubber spatula enables the technologist to firmly hold a small breast on the film holder without catching a hand under the compression paddle). The patient must lean forward so that the abdomen is not in the way of the x-ray beam.

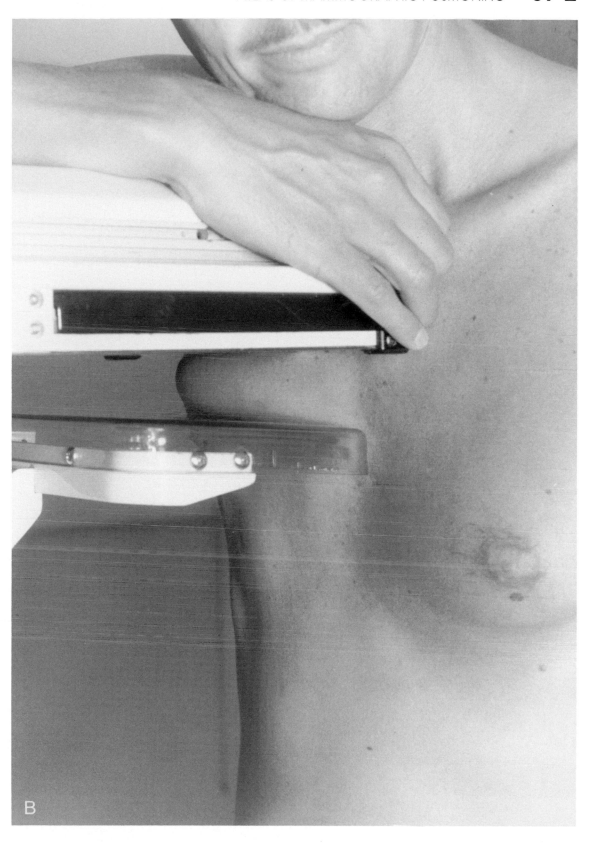

B

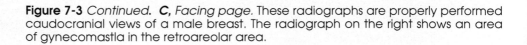

Figure 7-3 *Continued. C, Facing page.* These radiographs are properly performed caudocranial views of a male breast. The radiograph on the right shows an area of gynecomastla in the retroareolar area.

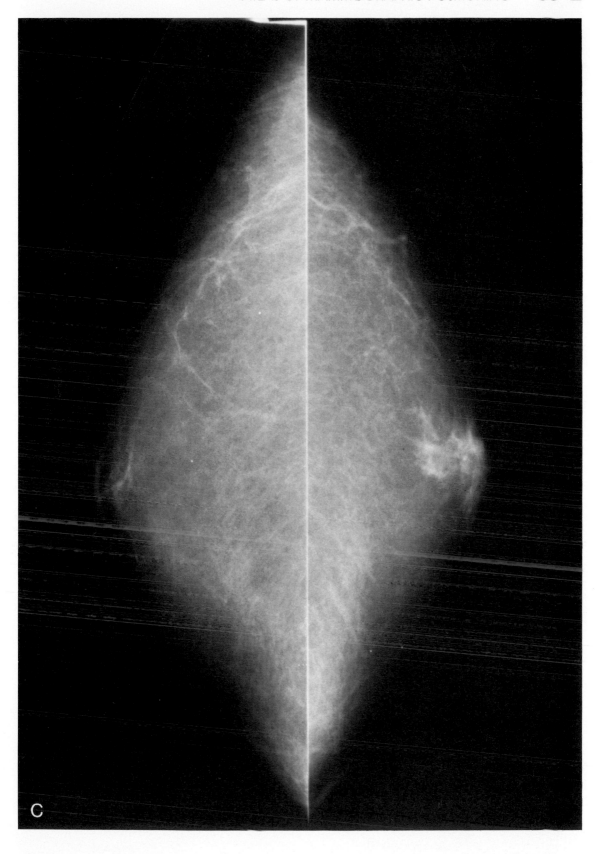

C

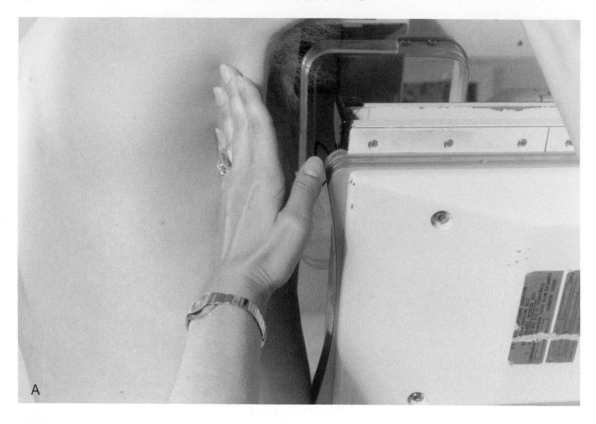

A

Figure 7-4. _A,_ A 65° tube angle is needed to match that of the pectoral muscle. The technologist must raise the C-arm so that the corner of the film goes into the hollow of the patient's axilla. In this figure the technologist shows the latissimus dorsi muscle that is to be placed behind the edge of the cassette holder.

   **B,** Top, facing page. The corner of the cassette holder is firmly placed in the hollow of the patient's axilla with the pectoral muscle in front and the latissimus dorsi muscle behind.

   **C,** Bottom, facing page. The technologist must use the mobile lateral border, as with any patient, and then use the up-and-out maneuver to spread the breast tissue onto the film holder as compression is engaged.

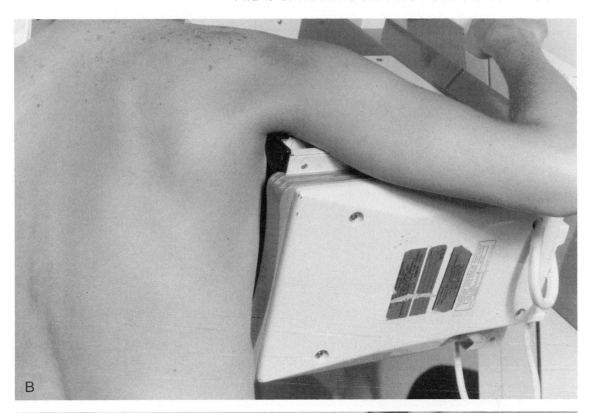

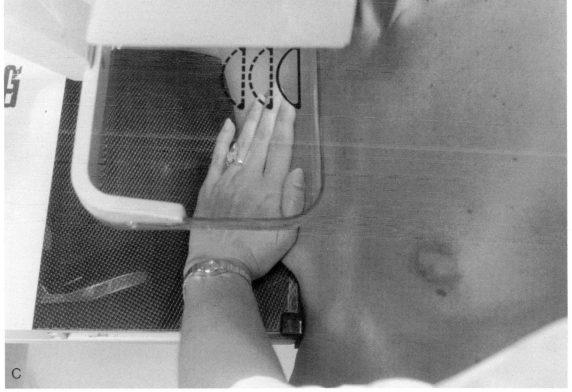

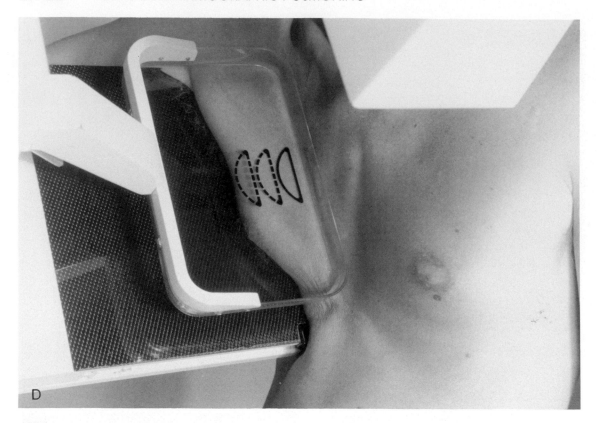

D

Figure 7-4 *Continued*. ***D***, This figure shows a mediolateral oblique view when properly positioned. Notice that the superior edge of the compression paddle is just below the head of the patient's humerus. The breast has been pulled straight out onto the film holder and the inframammary fold has been opened by pulling abdominal tissue down.

E, *Facing page.* These are properly positioned mediolateral oblique radiographs of a male breast. The radiograph on the left shows a small area of gynecomastia in the retroareolar area. A large portion of pectoral muscle is seen on both mediolateral obliques. Several lymph nodes are visualized in the pectoral area bilaterally.

There has been a reluctance in the past to compress the augmented breast for fear of damaging the implant and causing pain to the patient. Imaging the augmented breast presents a challenge to the technologist and requires special skills. A modified positioning technique has been developed for patients with implants. Displacing the implant posteriorly against the chest wall and pulling breast tissue over and in front of the implant results in an improvement in compression and the imaging of substantially more breast tissue.

Patient education for this procedure is paramount to ensure complete cooperation of the patient.

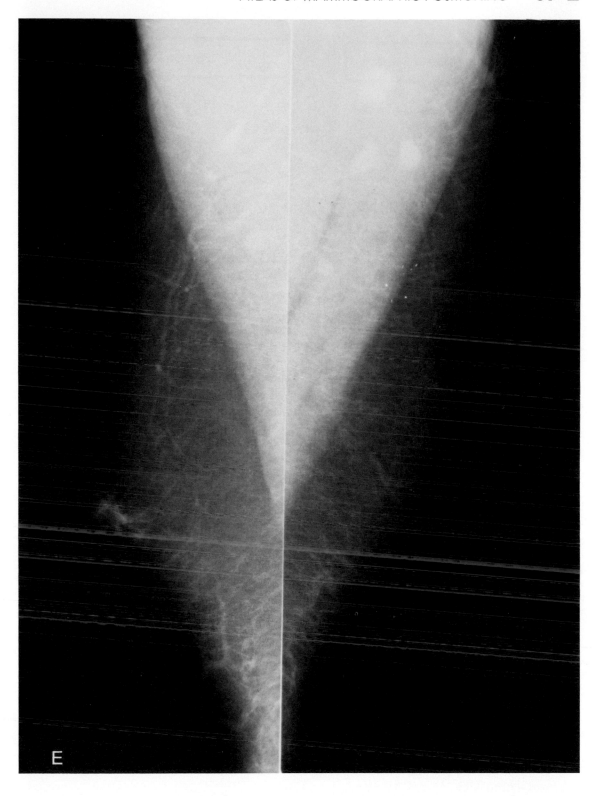

E

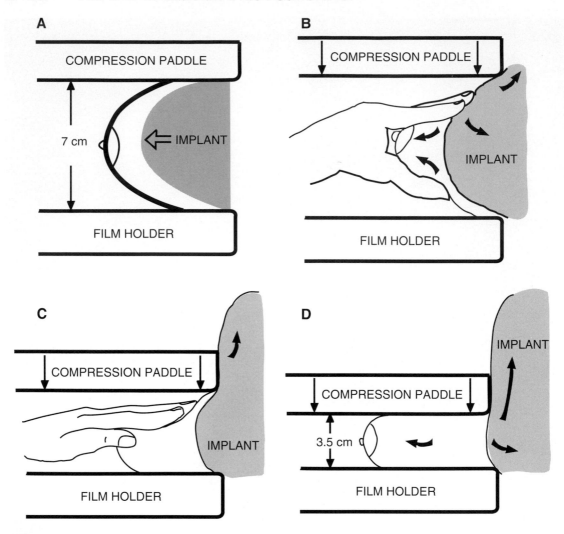

Figure 7-5. This figure shows the basic technique for the Eklund modified compression views (implant displaced). **A,** Compressing breast tissue together with an implant results in the implant's being driven forward, compacting the breast tissue and significantly limiting the degree of compression.

   B, C, Modified compression views begin with pulling of the breast tissue over and in front of the implant, while the technologist's hand and the compression paddle push the implant posteriorly as breast tissue is compressed.

   D, Breast tissue has been brought forward onto the film holder with compression displacing the implant posteriorly and excluding it from the field. (Reprinted from Eklund C W, Busby R C, et al.: Improved imaging of the augmented breast. AJR 151:469, 1988.)

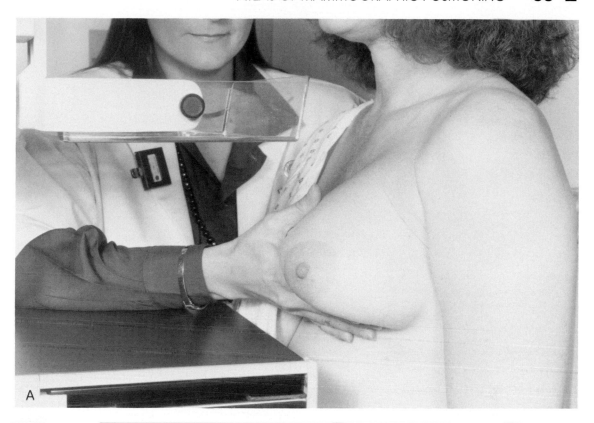

A

Figure 7-6. **A,** To begin the mammographic examination of a patient with breast implants, a routine craniocaudal view must be performed. In this figure the technologist is raising the patient's inframammary fold while standing on the medial side of the breast to be examined. The film holder will then be raised to meet the elevated level of the inframammary fold.

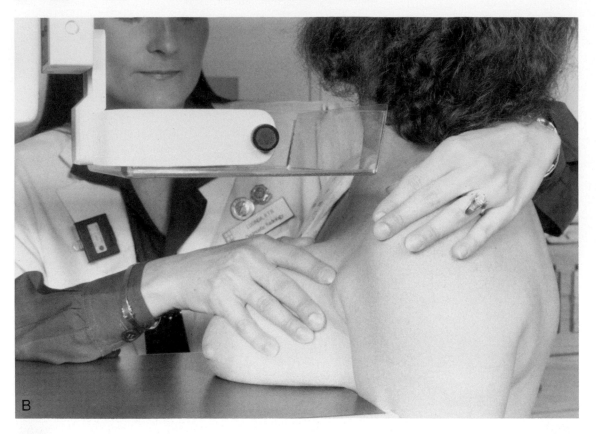

B

Figure 7-6 *Continued.* **B,** The technologist should relax the patient's shoulder down and forward with one hand while gently pulling the patient's entire breast forward onto the film with the other hand as compression is engaged.

C, *Facing page.* Before making the exposure, the technologist supinates the patient's entire arm to help eliminate skin folds on the lateral portion of the breast. This view requires a manually set exposure factor because the implant overlies the photosensor cell. Compression should be firm to eliminate motion unsharpness, but will be limited by the compressibility of the implant.

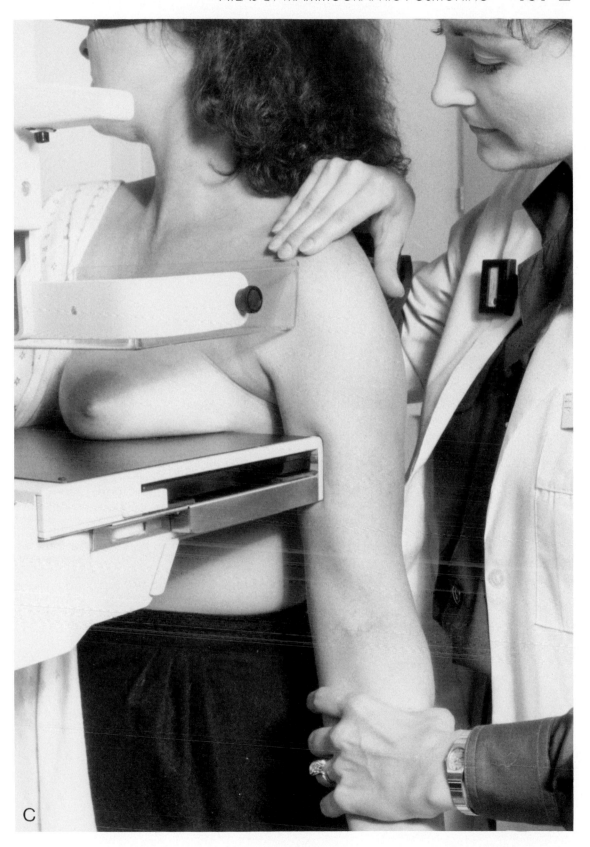

C

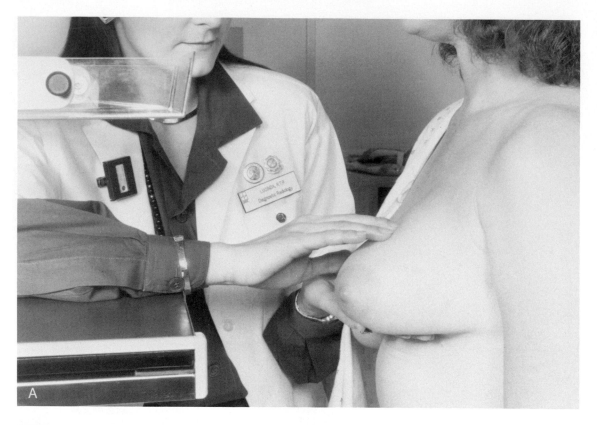

Figure 7-7. *A, Above,* Prior to displacing the implant for the modified craniocaudal view, the technologist should examine the patient. This enables the technologist to feel the firmness of the implant and determine how readily breast tissue may be displaced from it.

B, Top, facing page. Using both hands, the technologist grasps the patient's breast with the fingers on top and the thumbs below near the chest wall, gently pulling the superior and inferior breast tissue forward over the implant as well as all of the anterior tissue. The technologist becomes more efficient at this maneuver with practice.

C, Bottom, facing page. Once the breast tissue has been displaced anteriorly to the implant, the technologist places that part of the breast onto the film holder. The technologist must continue to hold the breast firmly in place or the implant will push forward, requiring that the view be restarted.

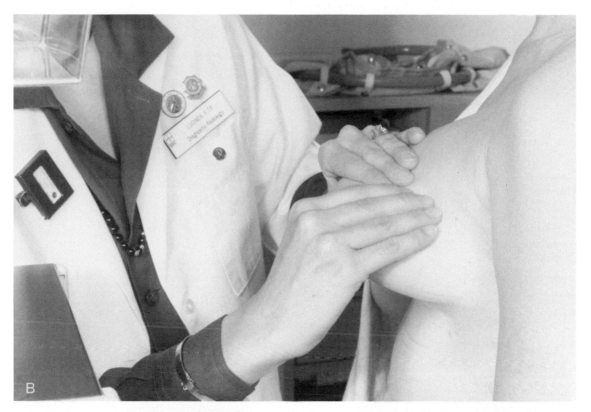

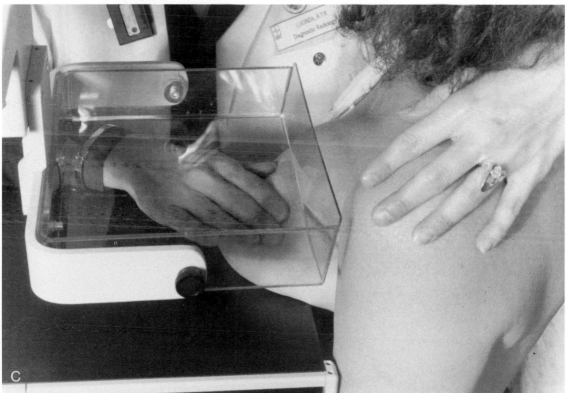

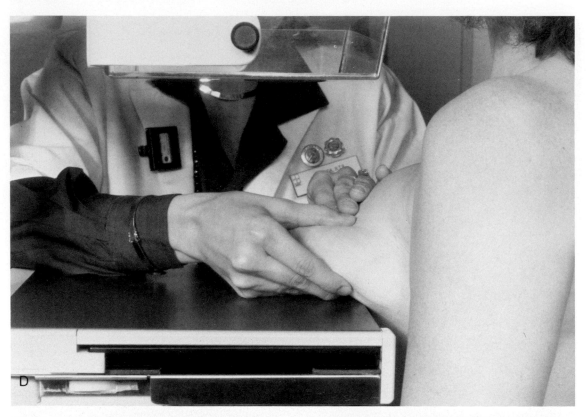

D

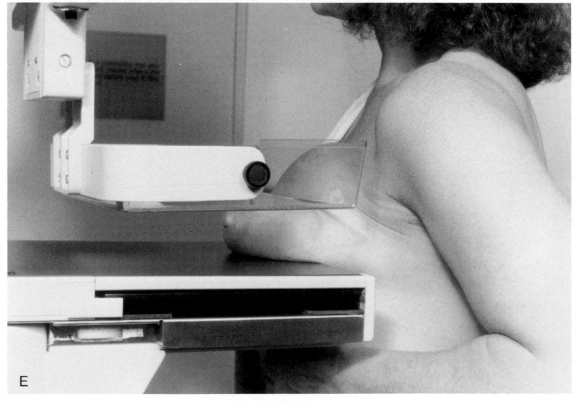

E

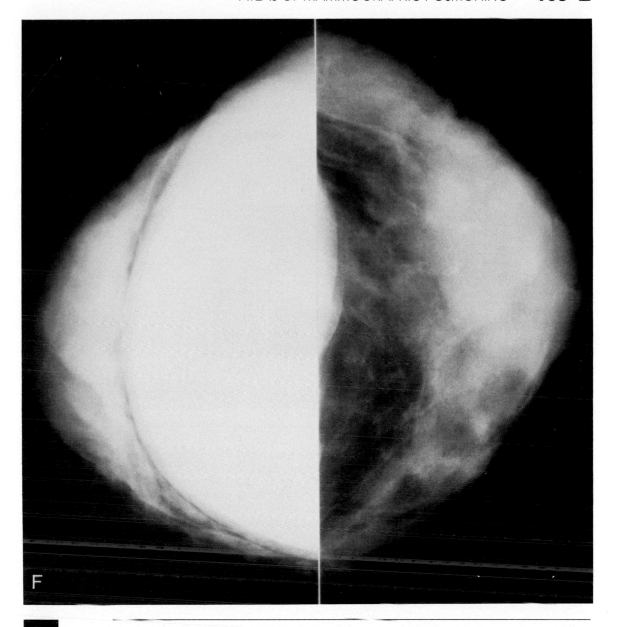

F

Figure 7-7 *Continued.* **D,** *Top, facing page.* As compression is engaged, the technologist can use her fingers on one hand to help spread the patient's breast tissue forward onto the film holder while using the other hand to hold the patient in place and keep her shoulder relaxed, down, and forward.

E, *Bottom, facing page.* This figure shows what the view looks like prior to exposure. The breast tissue has been pulled anteriorly forward onto the film holder and is adequately compressed while the implant has been displaced posteriorly against the chest wall. To steady the patient, the technologist may wish to have the patient place a hand between her abdomen and the film holder, where a natural space occurs for this view.

F, *Above.* The radiograph on the left is a properly compressed image of the breast and the undisplaced implant. This view best images breast tissue in the far medial and lateral areas. The radiograph on the right shows a properly positioned and compressed breast with the implant displaced (ID). A small amount of implant is visible in the field posteriorly.

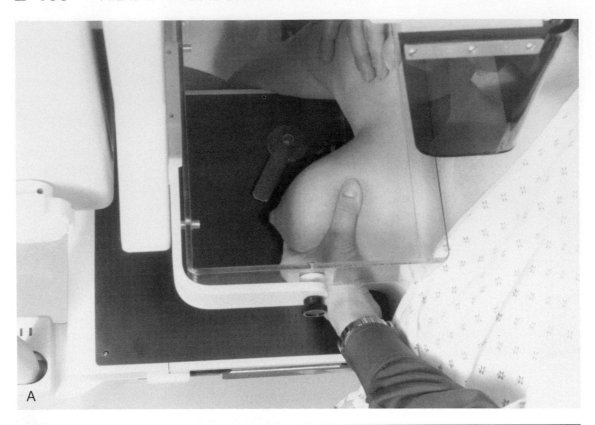

A

Figure 7-8. A, The technologist should begin the standard mediolateral oblique (MLO) view by choosing the correct angle of the pectoral muscle. The technologist places the hollow of the axilla on the superior corner of the film holder and makes sure that the patient's rib cage is firmly against it. The technologist pulls the patient's breast medially and rotates the patient down onto the film holder at the same time. As compression is engaged, the technologist guards the head of the humerus and clavicle, easing the skin up and over this area.

B, *Top, facing page.* The technologist uses the up-and-out maneuver with her hand to help hold the patient's breast tissue forward onto the film and away from the chest wall.

C, *Bottom, facing page.* It is important to use firm compression to reduce motion unsharpness, but the degree of compression that can be used is limited by the firmness of the implant. In this figure the technologist shows that breast tissue anterior to the implant is uncompressed.

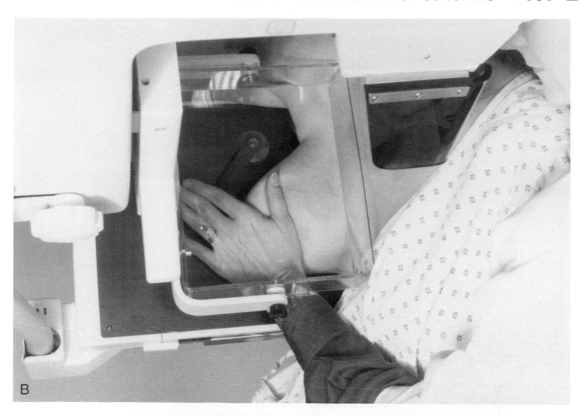

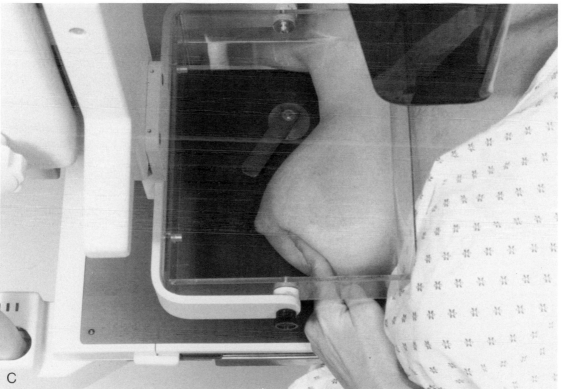

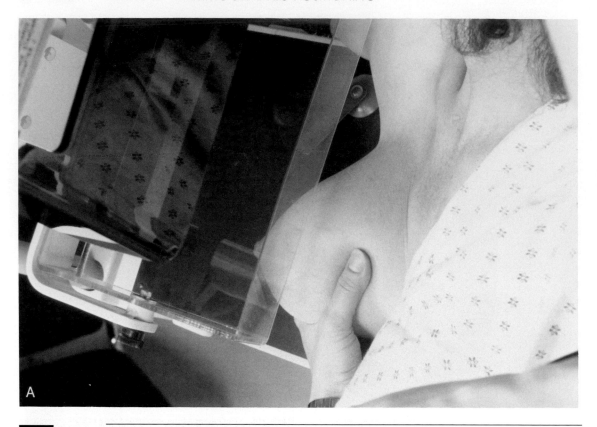

Figure 7-9. A, With the modified mediolateral oblique view, the technologist once again guides the hollow of the patient's axilla onto the superior corner of the film holder while pulling the patient's superomedial and inferolateral breast tissue forward along with anterior breast tissue in front of the implant. The technologist accomplishes this by grasping the patient's breast along the inferior surface with the palm of the hand. The technologist places her fingers against the lateral border and thumb on the medial breast tissue.

B, *Top, facing page.* Once this maneuver has been accomplished, the technologist rotates the patient down onto the film holder so that the lateral border of the patient's breast is placed firmly against the film holder. The technologist utilizes the up-and-out maneuver while compression is engaged.

C, *Bottom, facing page.* This figure shows what the position looks like prior to the radiographic exposure. The compression paddle has the implant pushed against the chest wall, allowing for better compression of breast tissue anterior to it. Notice that there is a small amount of pectoral muscle positioned on the cassette holder, but there is no inframammary fold.

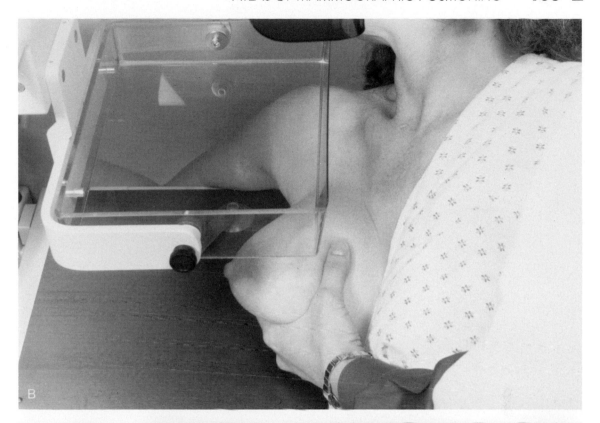

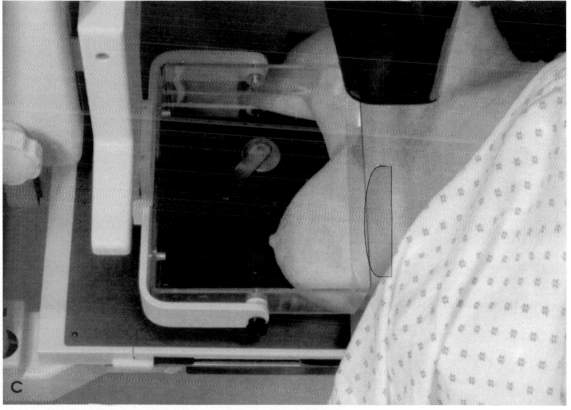

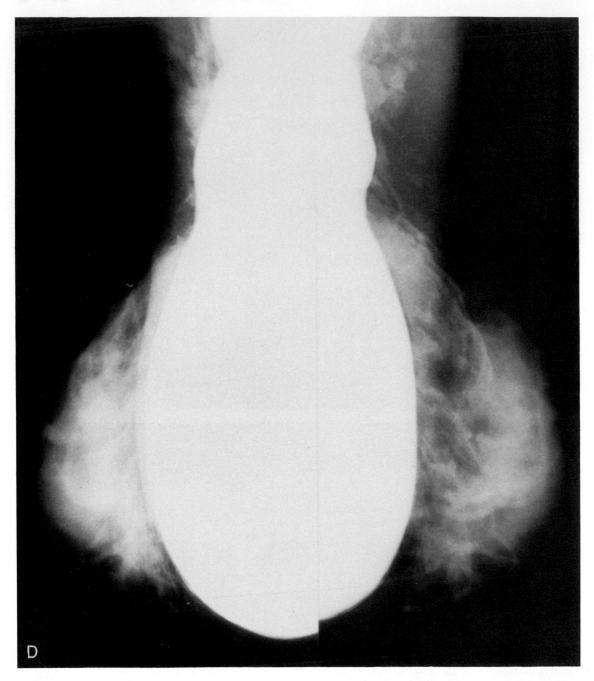

D

Figure 7-9 *Continued.* **D,** The radiograph on the left is a standard mediolateral oblique view that includes the implant. The implant limits the degree of compression and results in compacting of breast tissue between the implant and skin. The radiograph on the right is of the same patient after the technologist used the implant displaced (ID) technique. Moderate improvement in compression enables improved image detail. It is important to mention that the modified compression technique allows 2 cm to 5 cm of additional breast compression with little or no implant imaged in the field of interest.

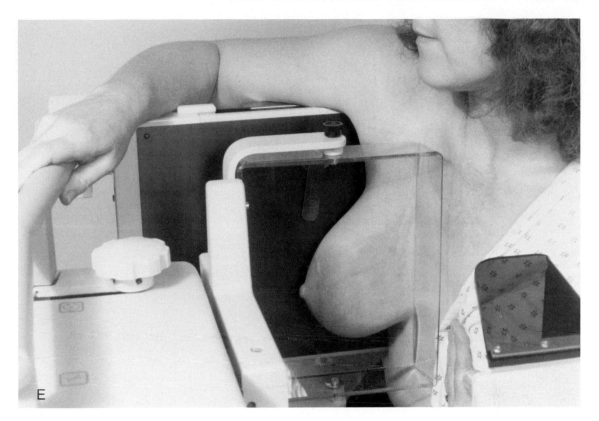

E

Figure 7-9 *Continued. E,* Patients whose breast implant has undergone rigid encapsulation will need an additional 90° lateral projection to provide imaging of the posterior breast tissue immediately above and below the implant. The projection is needed because the modified compression technique will not image breast tissue that remains posteriorly around the periphery of the implant.

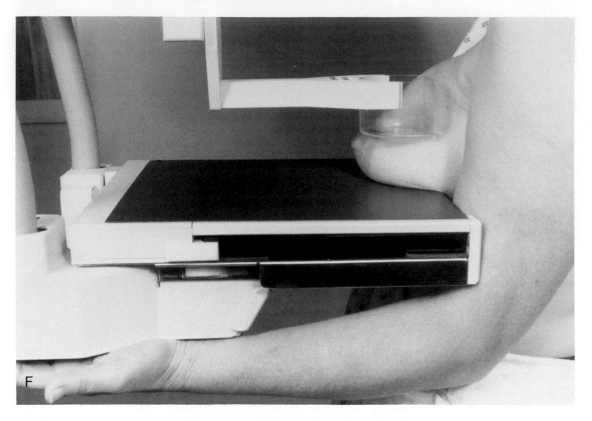

Figure 7-9 *Continued.* **F,** Spot compression with or without magnification may also be performed on patients with augmentation. The spot compression paddle is engaged while breast tissue is pulled over and in front of the implant, compressing only breast tissue whenever possible. This also enables the photosensor to be used.

CHAPTER EIGHT

Preoperative Needle Localization

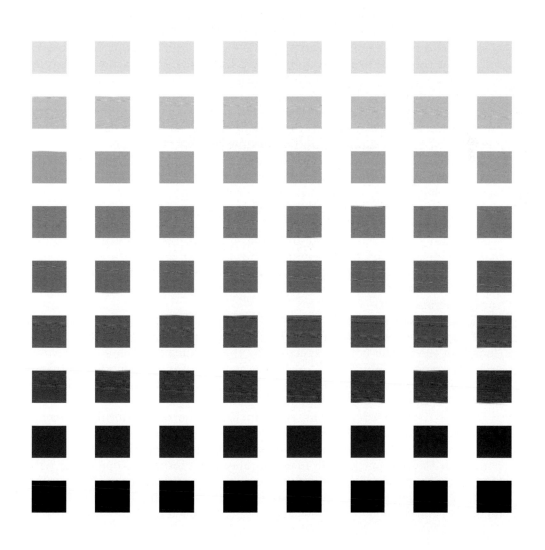

Using mammographic guidance, radiologists are able to localize clinically occult lesions. Precise needle placement is mandatory to guide surgical biopsy, ensure that the lesion is excised, and minimize the cosmetic defect. There are several approaches used for needle or wire localization of occult breast lesions. Patient safety, the accuracy of the procedure for the radiologist, and the approach of the surgeon must be taken into consideration when determining the best approach to take.

Institutions vary in their policies regarding who is responsible for explaining the preoperative needle localization procedure to the patient. The technologist must make sure that the patient fully understands the procedure before she is placed on the mammographic unit. Patient cooperation is critical to the success of the preoperative needle placement.

PREPARATION

Local anesthesia (1 percent lidocaine) may be used although it is not always needed. Many women feel that the administration of the local anesthesia is more painful than the preoperative needle localization. If the patient and the radiologist choose to use local anesthesia, a history of the patient's allergies must be taken to help ensure that the patient does not have an adverse reaction to the anesthesia. It is important that general anesthesia (sedation) not be given to the patient prior to preoperative needle placement, for the patient must be clear-headed and able to follow instructions. Once the patient has been placed on the mammographic machine for the exam, she should never be left alone in the room. Many patients experience a high level of anxiety, and a vasovagal reaction, although infrequent, may occur. The radiologist or the technologist may want to distract the patient with pleasant conversation to help soothe her nerves and also prevent her from viewing the needle, which can be frightening. If the patient experiences a vasovagal reaction, the technologist should remove her from the machine (being careful not to dislodge the needle), and have her lie supine with her legs up for several minutes. This is normally all that is required for a quick recovery, after which the procedure may be completed. Medication is rarely needed to treat a vasovagal reaction.

The preoperative needle placement is done under sterile conditions, so a prep tray is needed. Included on the tray are 1) a breast localization needle (length of the needle is to be specified by the radiologist); 2) a 1.0-cc syringe and a 25-gauge needle if local anesthesia is to be used; 3) some form of povidone-iodine swab sticks for cleansing the skin; 4) steristrips for taping the needle or wire to the skin; and 5) sterile gauze sponges.

Other items needed in the room include 1 percent lidocaine, alcohol wipes, sterile gloves, and nonsterile tape. The equipment used for the mammographic examination must be a dedicated mammographic unit. A special paddle on the mammographic machine may have either an open hole with lead markers on two sides for determination of coordinates or multiple holes. If a multiple-hole paddle is used, the technologist should make sure that the hole size is large enough to allow clearance of the needle hub.

CHOICE OF THE LOCALIZATION GUIDE

The choice of the localization guide is made by the radiologist and the surgeon based on where the area of interest lies in the patient's breast.

Hypodermic Needle

The simplest guide to use is a standard hypodermic needle with or without an injection of methylene blue. The advantages of using a hypodermic needle are that 1) the needle is stiff so that the surgeon can easily palpate its course, facilitating accurate surgery; 2) the needle can be easily removed and repositioned by the radiologist if the relationship to the lesion is incorrect. The disadvantages of using a hypodermic needle are that 1) because the needle hub sits above the skin, inadvertent snagging of the needle may cause it to be pulled out of the breast prematurely; and 2) a straight needle provides only two-dimensional accuracy. The surgeon must estimate the distance of the lesion along the needle shaft.

Hook Wire Systems

Hook wire systems include the Kopans spring hook wire, the Homer curved end wire, and the Hawkins-retractable barb wire. The advantages of a hook wire system are that 1) wires offer the most accurate three-dimensional localization, and 2) wires are flexible and may be anchored securely to the skin, making it difficult for them to become dislodged. The disadvantages of a hook wire system are that 1) most often the surgeon will need to follow the wire directly from the skin insertion site into the breast, and the wire may be difficult to locate in breast tissue; 2) wires may not be used by surgeons as retractors because with sufficient traction they may be pulled out of the breast; if they are located in fat instead of in fibroglandular tissue, the wire has a tendency to move; and 3) the wire must be long enough so that it will not be pulled into the breast when compression is released and the breast is in its natural position. This is especially important when used in a large pendulous breast or when the patient is supine for the procedure.

ANTEROPOSTERIOR APPROACH

Two approaches are most often used for the preoperative needle placement. The first, the anteroposterior approach, introduces the needle from the front of the breast. The radiologist measures the distance of the lesion from the nipple in two projections (the craniocaudal and the 90° lateral views). These measurements are then transposed from the mammogram to the uncompressed breast. The initial placement of an anteroposterior guide is an approximation because of the elasticity of the breast and the variable magnification seen on the mammogram. Orthogonal mammograms must be obtained to estimate the relationship and distance of the needle tip from the lesion. The needle may then be repositioned for a more accurate placement with additional orthogonal mammograms obtained to confirm accuracy. The needle may be repositioned several times before it is in the desired relationship to the lesion.

The advantage of the anteroposterior approach is that many surgeons prefer the needle or wire to be placed in this position to facilitate surgery because it parallels the surgical approach. A periareolar incision may be used if the needle is inserted at the areolar limbus. This incision results in a scar that is more cosmetically acceptable. The disadvantages of the anteroposterior approach are that 1) the anteroposterior approach cannot be done under direct visualization because mammograms can be obtained only orthogonal to this direction; 2) this procedure is operator-dependent, requiring the ability of the operator to triangulate; and 3) an anteroposterior approach may be suited for only superficial lesions. With lesions close to the chest wall, caution is strongly advised so that the needle is not inserted into the pectoral muscle or through it into the pleural space, lung, or mediastinum. A pneumothorax may be caused by introducing needles in this direction during the localization of deep breast lesions. If the patient is supine for the procedure and the wire is too short for the depth of the lesion, the wire may disappear into the breast as the patient sits up. Not only have wires retracted into the breast, but some of those wires that were not immediately retrieved have eventually passed into other body parts.

THE PARALLEL APPROACH

The second needle placement plane and approach of choice is parallel to the chest wall. Many localization complications can be avoided with this technique. In this approach, the shortest measurement usually dictates the approach to the lesion. The movement is found through the use of two preliminary films, a craniocaudal view and a 90° lateral view. The craniocaudal view measures the distance from the lesion to the lateral or medial skin surface. The 90° view, whether medial or lateral, measures the distance from the lesion to the superior or inferior skin surface. For example, if the lesion is closest to the medial surface of the breast on the craniocaudal view, needle positioning is accomplished in a 90° mediolateral approach with the needle inserted from the medial skin surface. If the lesion is close to the lateral surface of the breast in the craniocaudal view, a 90° lateromedial approach is used. A lesion near the top of the breast in a 90° lateral view is localized by utilizing a craniocaudal projection. Similarly, a lesion seen at the bottom of the breast on a 90° lateral view is localized by using a caudocranial projection.

The advantages of the parallel approach are that 1) the most accurate method of positioning a needle for preoperative needle localization is through the use of orthogonal views, utilizing the parallel-to-chest wall approach: the breast is held in the compression paddle during the procedure with the lesion under direct visualization; 2) the procedure is easily mastered; and 3) the parallel approach is the safest method available. The disadvantages of the parallel approach are that 1) preoperative needle placement parallel to the chest wall is not always ideal for the surgical approach, because many surgeons prefer to use an incision from a circumareolar incision, dissecting from the needle or wire directly back toward the chest wall; and 2) from the radiologist's viewpoint, parallel-to-chest wall needle placement from a caudocranial (FB) view is awkward and may be uncomfortable for the patient.

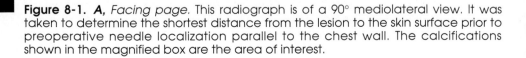

Figure 8-1. A, *Facing page.* This radiograph is of a 90° mediolateral view. It was taken to determine the shortest distance from the lesion to the skin surface prior to preoperative needle localization parallel to the chest wall. The calcifications shown in the magnified box are the area of interest.

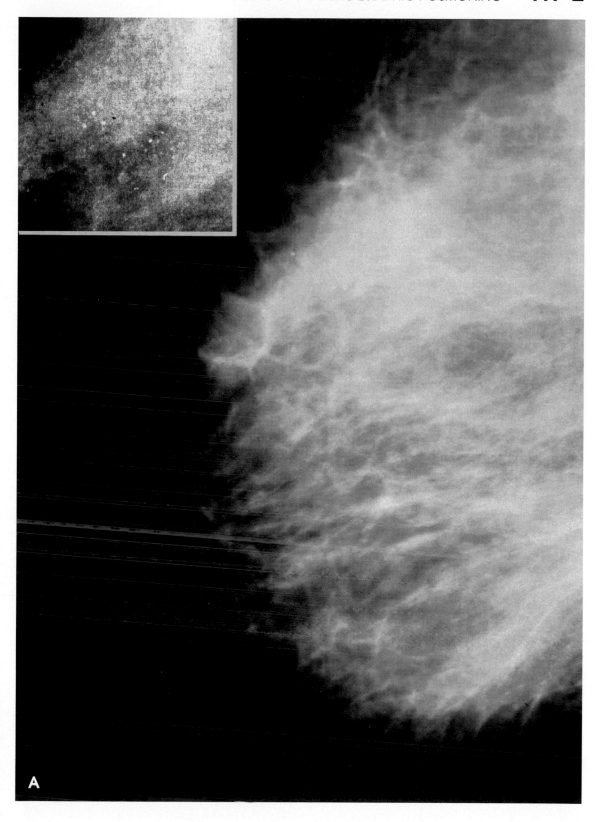

A

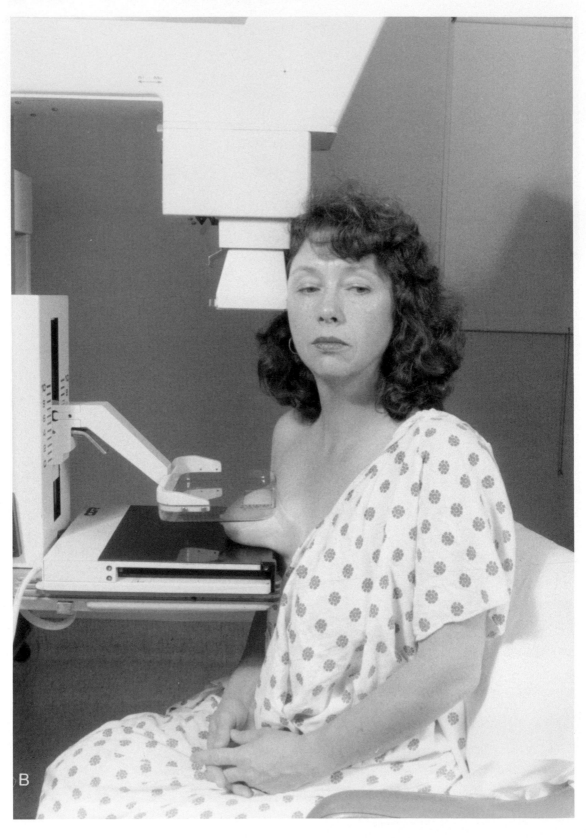

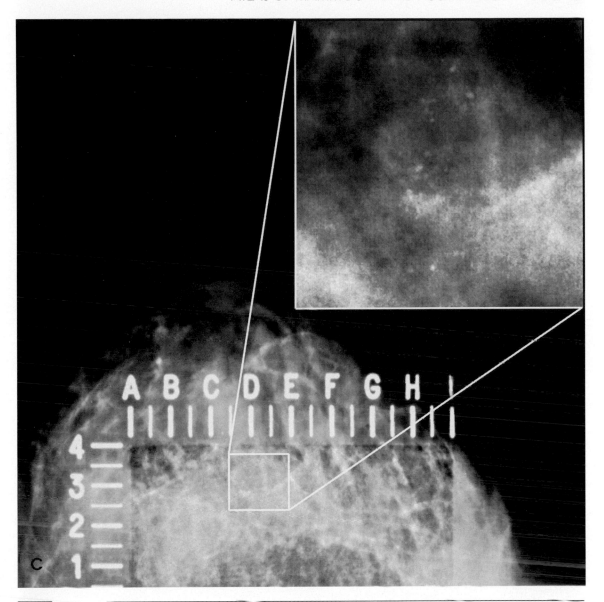

Figure 8-1 *Continued.* **B,** *Facing page.* The shortest distance has been determined and the patient is placed with her breast compressed in a fenestrated compression paddle. The patient should be made as comfortable as possible once she is seated in this position. In this figure, the patient has been given back support with a pillow. If the room is chilly, the technologist may want to wrap the patient's legs in a blanket. If the chair the patient is sitting in has wheels, it is important that the wheels be securely locked for patient safety and to prevent subtle movement of the body during the procedure.

C, *Above.* Once the preliminary mammogram has been taken, the area of interest should lie within the opening of the compression paddle.

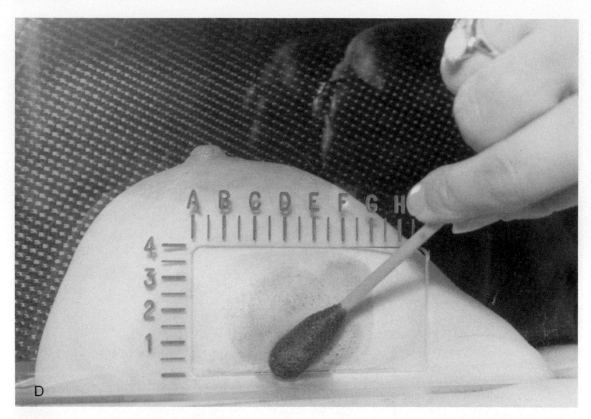

D

Figure 8-1 *Continued.* **D,** The skin should be thoroughly cleaned with povidone before the needle is introduced.

E, Top, facing page. The X and Y coordinates are determined from the marks around the opening of the compression paddle. These coordinates can be correlated with those on the preliminary radiograph.

F, Bottom, facing page. This figure shows the point at which the needle is introduced.

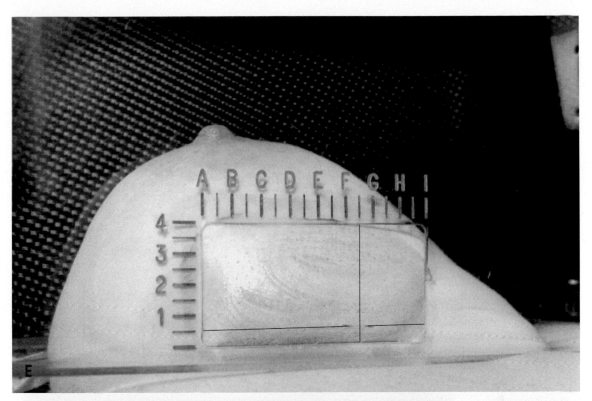

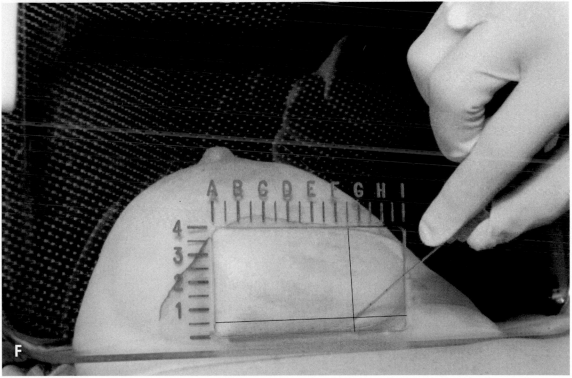

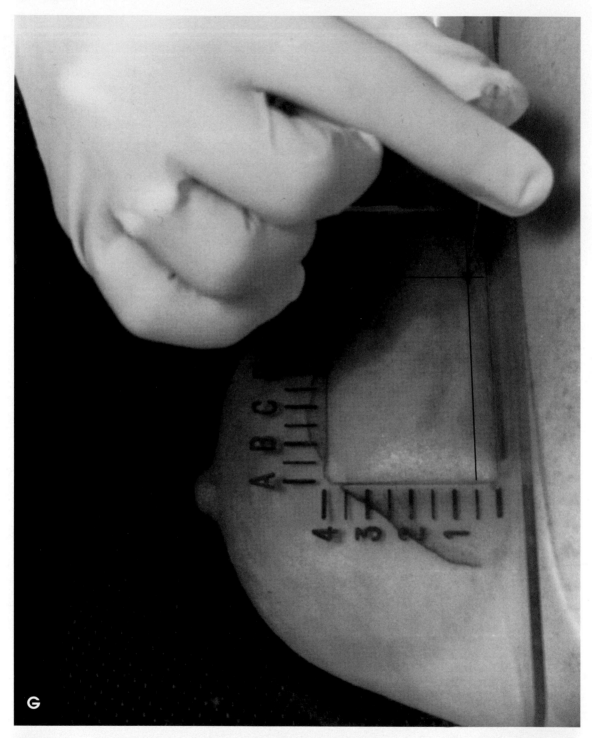

G

Figure 8-1 *Continued.* **G,** As the needle advances, its hub (top) should be superimposed on the shaft of the needle itself. This can be accomplished by using the centering light on the mammography unit. The x-ray beam and lights are generally aligned; if the shadow of the hub superimposes on the needle shaft under the light field with the tip directly over the lesion, the needle will be properly aligned on the mammogram.

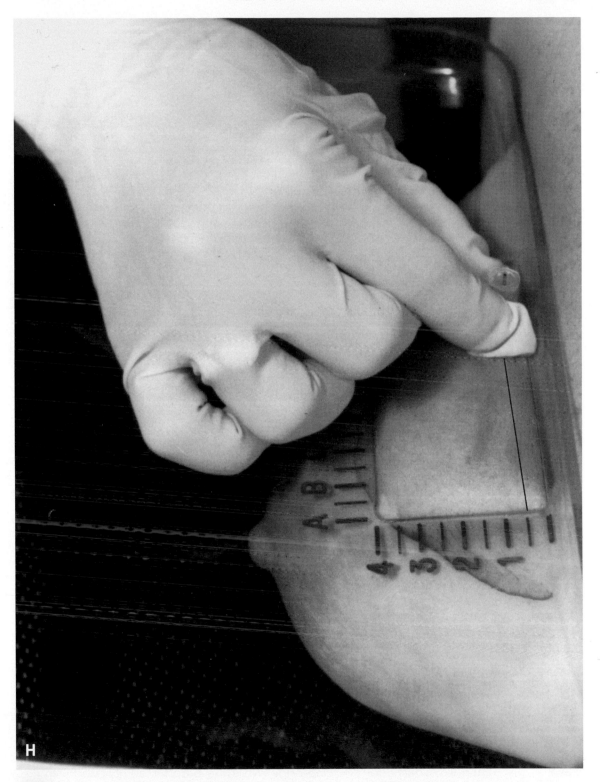

H

Figure 8-1 *Continued.* *H,* The needle will be advanced so that its hub goes to the skin line. This will ensure that the tip of the needle passes through the suspicious lesion it is impaling.

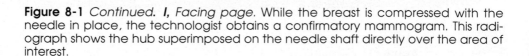

Figure 8-1 *Continued.* *I, Facing page.* While the breast is compressed with the needle in place, the technologist obtains a confirmatory mammogram. This radiograph shows the hub superimposed on the needle shaft directly over the area of interest.

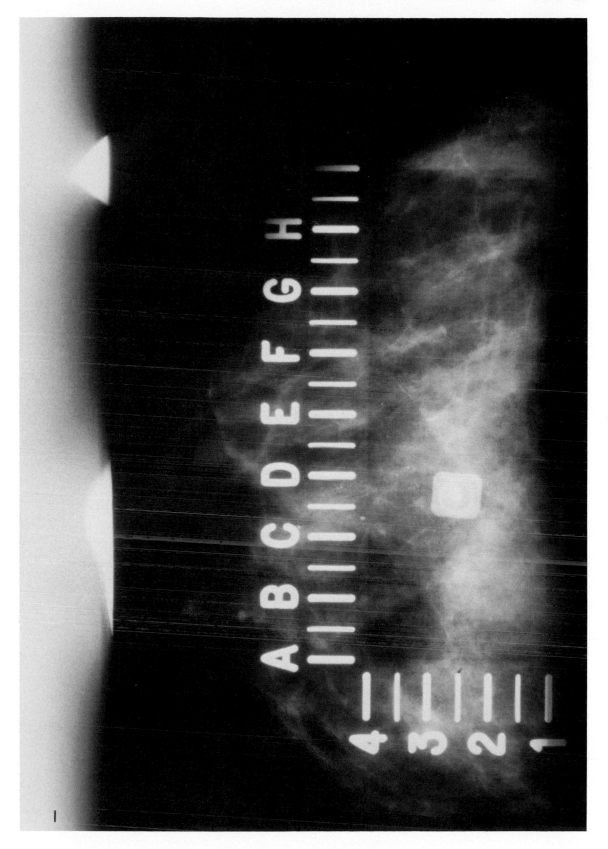

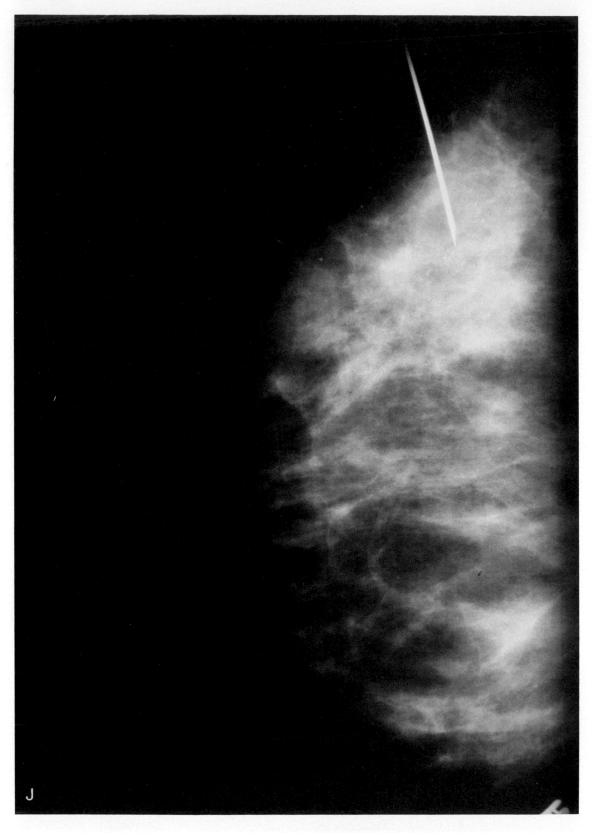

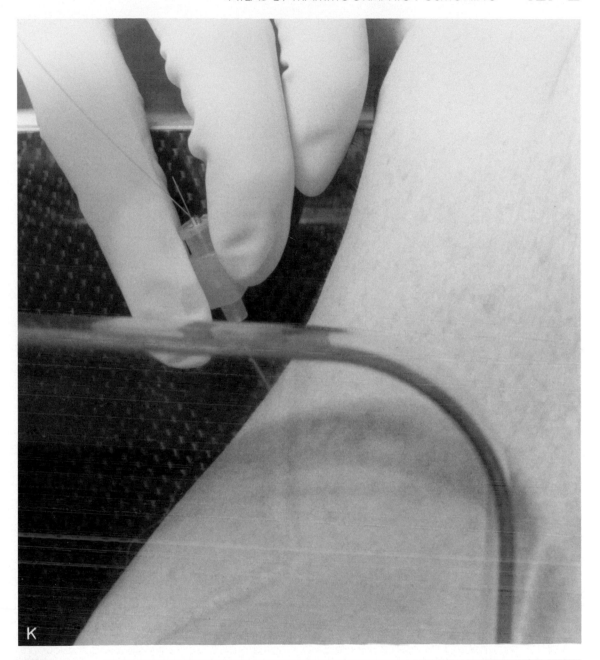

K

Figure 8-1 *Continued.* **J,** *Facing page.* Once the radiologist has achieved an accurate position in one plane, the technologist releases the compression paddle and moves the patient away from the mammographic unit. The machine's C-arm must be rotated to 90° for a true lateral projection. This projection will determine the depth of the needle tip. This view may be obtained either with a spot compression device over the area of interest or with a full compression paddle, depending on the preference of the radiologist. This radiograph shows a 90° mediolateral view with full compression. The tip of the needle is directly over the area of interest. If simple needle technique is used, this orthogonal projection is the final view required.

   K, *Above.* In this figure, a hook wire system is being used for localization. The wire will be advanced through the shaft to the tip of the needle, where it will spring open and be securely hooked into the breast tissue.

■

Figure 8-1 *Continued.* ***L,*** *Facing page.* Once the hook wire has been engaged, the needle may be safely removed, leaving only the wire protruding from the skin.

M, *Page 130.* This radiograph is of a 90° mediolateral view with the hook wire marking the area to be biopsied. Once the radiologist is satisfied with the location of the wire, the patient may be released from the mammographic unit. The technologist securely fastens the end of the wire to the patient's skin using Steri-Strips. This prevents the wire from migrating deeper into the patient's breast away from the area of interest. Gauze padding may be taped over the entire area to keep it protected and clean.

N, *Page 131.* After the surgical biopsy, specimen radiography will be performed to make sure that the area of interest is located within the specimen. Magnification of the compressed specimen allows imaging of small masses as well as of calcifications. This figure shows a specimen radiograph of the excised breast tissue. Calcifications can be seen in the specimen at the tip of the hook wire. The pathology report showed this specimen to be not a carcinoma but sclerosing adenosis.

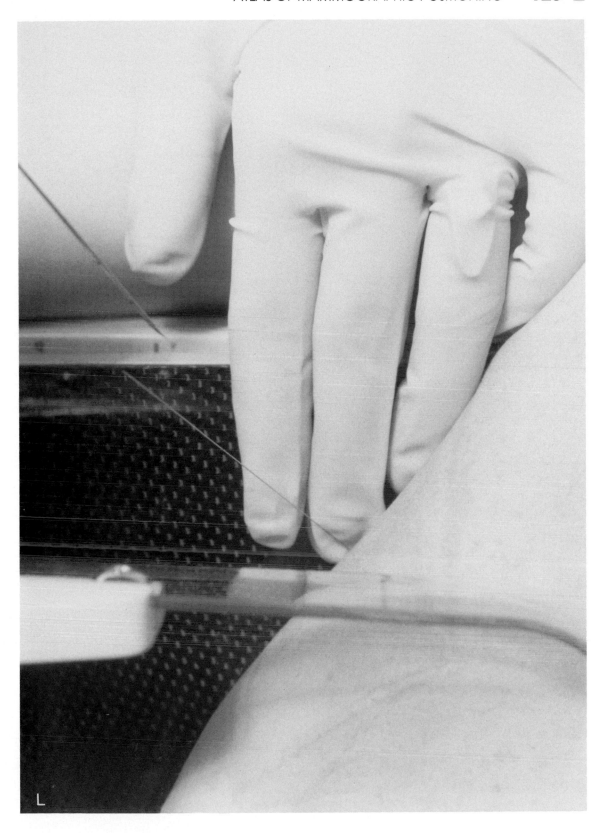

L

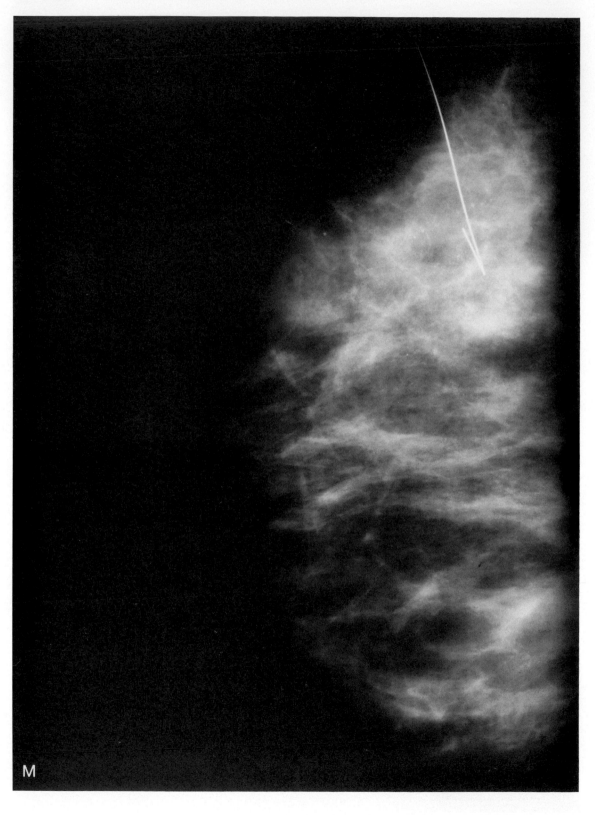

M

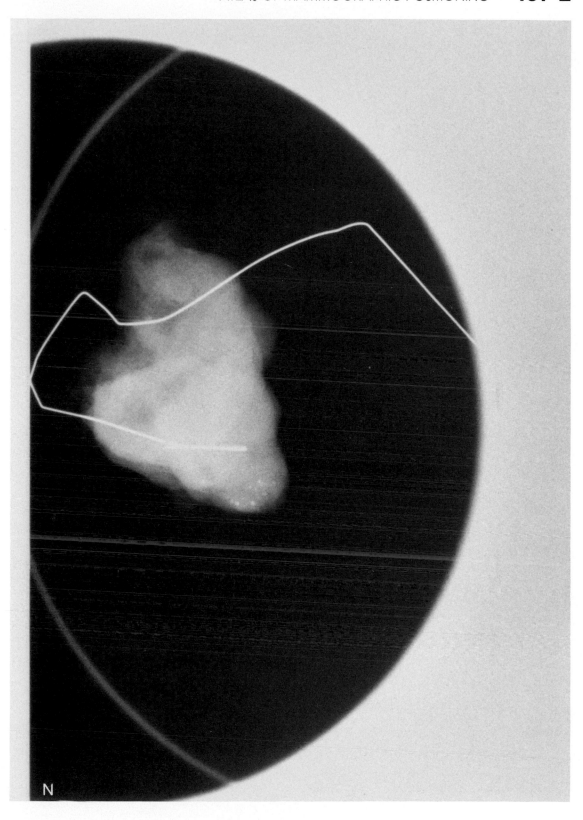

N

CHAPTER NINE

Patient History and the Clinical Breast Examination

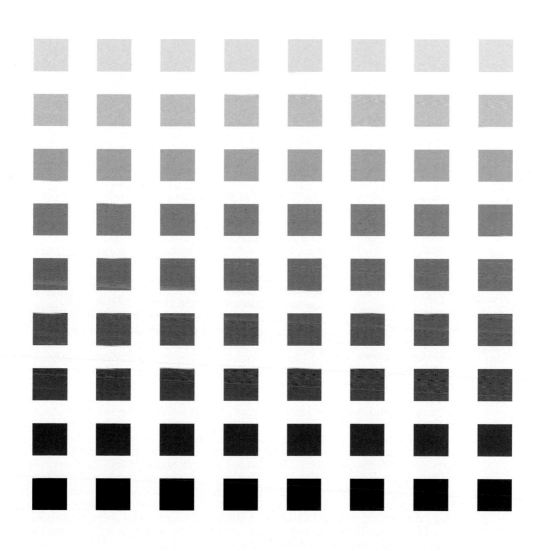

The technologist's role in the mammographic suite has been expanding over the last several years. Not only is the technologist concerned with producing a high quality mammogram, but she is also responsible for obtaining a thorough history from every patient. In many facilities, that history may include a visual inspection of the breast, as well as clinical palpation to correlate any problems the patient may be having. This chapter discusses 1) the importance of a thorough patient history; 2) the visual inspection of the breast; and 3) how to perform a clinical breast examination.

■

Figure 9-1. A, *Facing page.* It is important for the patient to fully understand the need for the technologist to obtain a complete patient history. The radiologist uses this information to correlate with his or her findings on the mammogram and to recommend guidelines for follow-up care.

B, *Pages 136–137.* This is a standard information sheet. Screening mammography is not normally recommended for patients under age 35, so asking the patient's age and birthdate is necessary. The technologist also must find out if the patient is experiencing a breast problem that may dictate the need for extra mammographic views. Any symptoms should be documented. The technologist obtains both family and personal history from the patient to help the radiologist correlate the risk factors of breast cancer for each patient. If the patient has been treated for breast cancer, this information must be documented under the personal history; it will help the technologist to choose the appropriate technical factors for the mammographic examination of a patient who has undergone lumpectomy and radiation therapy. It is also helpful for the technologist to have knowledge of any other breast surgery, such as augmentation or reduction, because the mammographic technical factors will be different for these patients also. The patient's menstrual and pregnancy histories are also needed. In addition, a biopsy history is important because all scars must be documented so that the radiologist can correlate them with what he or she sees on the patient's mammogram. Certain medications may affect breast tissue. If the patient has been placed on female hormones since her last mammogram, documentation of this is important so that the radiologist will have a better understanding of possible changes on the current mammographic study. As stated previously, it is important to be able to compare the current study with any prior mammograms. If the patient does not bring her previous mammograms with her, it is necessary for her to sign a release form so that they may be obtained.

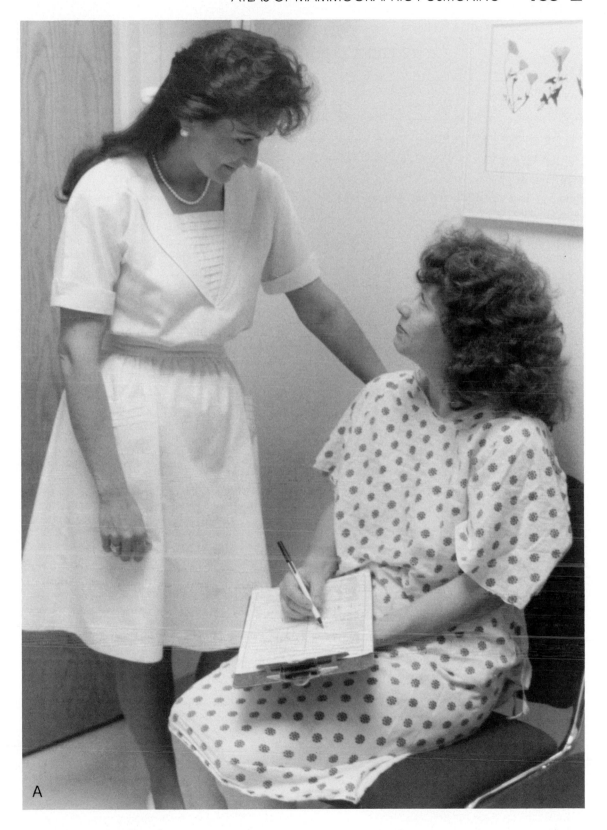

A

ID # _____

BSC _____
Screen only _____

PATIENT INFORMATION SHEET

NAME: _____ MED REC # _____

DATE: _____ NEW UW PATIENT?: ____ Yes ____ No

AGE: _____ SEX: _____ WEIGHT: _____ HEIGHT: _____

Who is your personal physician? _____

Who referred you here for today's exam/mammogram? _____

SYMPTOMS:

Have you had any of the following symptoms?
- ____ Lump or mass
  - ____ Found by me
  - ____ Found by health provider
  - Lump changes w/menstrual cycle?
  - ____ Yes ____ No ____ Don't know
- ____ Nipple discharge
- ____ Pain or tenderness
  - Pain changes w/menstrual cycle?
  - ____ Yes ____ No
- ____ Skin change
- ____ Change in appearance of nipple
- ____ Previous abnormal mammogram
- ____ Other _____
- ____ None, here for screening

X-RAY HISTORY:

Have you ever had a mammogram? ____Yes ____ No
Where? _____
Date of most recent _____

Have you ever had an abnormal mammogram?
____ Yes ____ No
When? _____
What kind of follow-up did you have?

_____

Have you ever had an ultrasound procedure on your breast? ____ Yes ____ No
Where? _____
Date of most recent _____

SURGERY HISTORY:

Have you ever had a breast biopsy? ____Yes ____No

Date	R/L	Surgical or Needle?	Diagnosis
____	____	____	_____
____	____	____	_____
____	____	____	_____
____	____	____	_____

Have you had any breast surgery? ____Yes ____No

Augmentation ____ Implants ____
Reduction ____ Cyst removal ____
Other _____

FAMILY/PERSONAL HISTORY:

Do you have a family history of breast cancer? ____Yes ____No
If yes, list age, relationship; note if maternal or paternal side:

_____

_____

_____

_____

Have you ever had breast cancer? ____Yes ____No
If yes, when? _____
Mark location on picture below with a circle:

Size when found _____
How was it discovered?
X-ray ____ MD ____ By me ____
Were lymph nodes involved? ____Yes ____No

Treatment:
None ____ Removal of lump ____
Mastectomy ____
Radiotherapy (dates) _____ to _____
Chemotherapy (dates) _____ to _____

Have you had any other cancer? ____Yes ____No
If yes, what kind? _____
When? _____

Have you had other breast disease? ____Yes ____No
Benign tumor or cyst ____ Fibrocystic disease ____
Infection ____ Other ____

Do you do monthly breast self-exams? ____Yes ____No

When was your last pelvic exam? _____
Pap smear _____
Breast exam _____

B

MENSTRUAL/PREGNANCY HISTORY:

Are you pregnant now? ____Yes ____No   Have you reached menopause? ____Yes ____No
If yes when _____

When was your last menstrual period? _____
Do you have regular periods? ____ Yes ____ No   Age at your first period _____

How many pregnancies have you had? _____
How many births? _____ Age at first pregnancy _____

Did you try to breastfeed? ____Yes ____ No
If yes, how many children? _____ How long? _____

Have you had a hysterectomy? ____ Yes ____ No   If yes, why? _____
Were your ovaries removed? ____Yes ____ No

Are you on any of the following medications now:

Birth control pills ____ Estrogen____ Progesterone ____
Tamoxifen ____ Thyroid medication____ Tranquilizers ____

Anti-depressants ____ Ulcer medication ____ Other _____

Have you ever taken female hormones? ____Yes ____ No   For how long? _____

When did you stop taking them? _____

How much caffeine do you drink a day? _____ (cups/cans)

How much alcohol do you drink in a week? _____

Do you use tobacco? ____Yes ____ No   If yes, what kind? _____ How much? _____

FOR CLINIC USE:

Disposition:

Mammogram ____Yes ____ No

Referred to UW Clinic? ____Yes ____ No   **If yes, where?** _____
                                            when? _____

Referred/recommended for pap/pelvic _____ **Other** _____

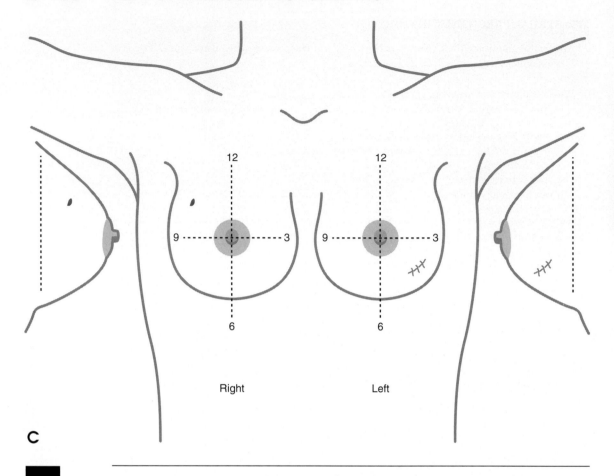

C

Figure 9-1 *Continued.* **C,** This patient information sheet may be used by the technologist to document abnormalities described by the patient as well as biopsy scars, skin lesions such as moles and keloids, or anything else that may project over the breast. Diagrams used for documentation should have a frontal as well as a lateral projection so that the technologist may indicate the distance of the abnormality from the nipple and its relationship to the chest wall. If one breast is larger than the other, the patient should be asked whether she has noticed the uneven breast sizes and the length of time she has been aware of the unevenness. On this diagram the technologist has indicated that there is a mole (•) at 10 o'clock, which is in the upper outer quadrant of the right breast, as well as a biopsy scar (⫫) located at 4 o'clock in the lower outer quadrant of the left breast. The technologist uses the face of a clock overlying the diagram of the breast to accurately describe the location of any markings on the skin to the radiologist.

THE 7 Ps

The American Cancer Society of California has developed a helpful technique for clinical breast examination called the "seven Ps." Following the 7 Ps helps the technologist to remember the components of complete clinical breast examination: 1) positions; 2) perimeter; 3) palpation technique with pads; 4) pressure; 5) pattern of search; 6) practice with feedback; and 7) plan of action.

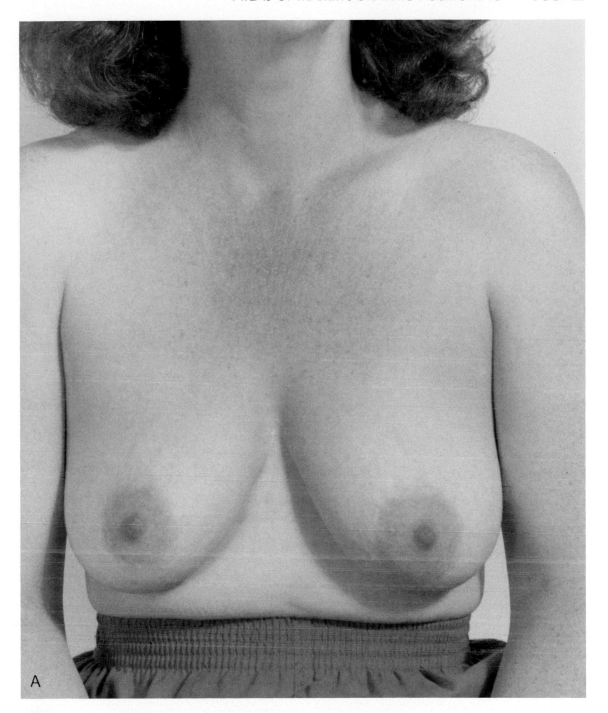

A

Figure 9-2. ***A*, Positions for visual inspection.** When performing a clinical breast examination, it is important to inspect the breasts under good lighting because subtle contour changes such as dimpling may otherwise be missed. The technologist begins the visual inspection with the patient seated. The patient's arms should be relaxed at her sides. The technologist looks for any change in size and shape from the right breast to the left. Skin changes such as redness, ulceration, or edema should be noted, as should other abnormalities including nipple deviation, retraction, or discharge.

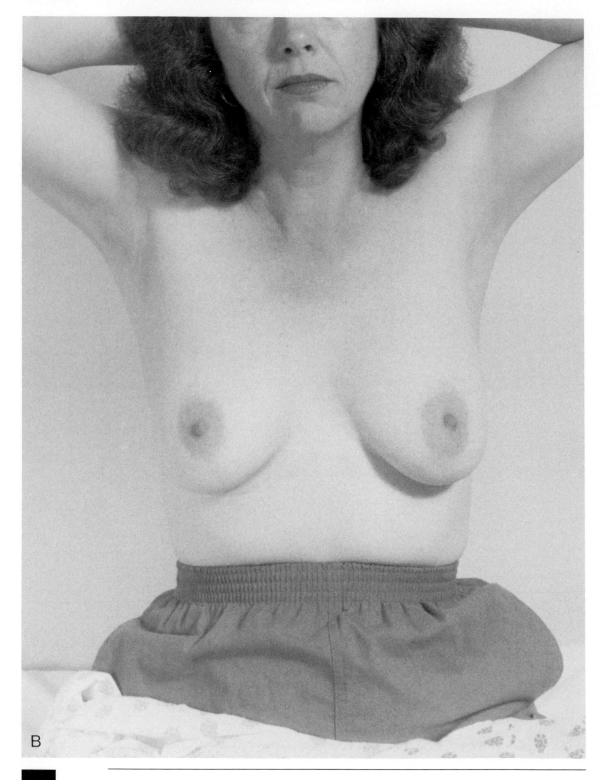

B

Figure 9-2 *Continued*. **B,** The technologist should have the patient raise her hands over her head to expose the undersides of both breasts. Once again, the technologist looks for dimpling or other skin abnormalities.

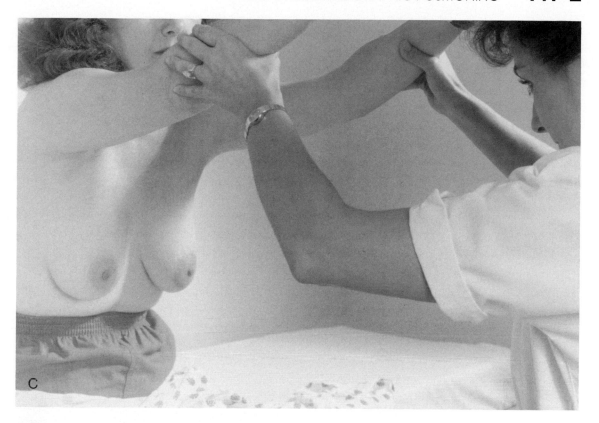

C

Figure 9-2 *Continued.* **C,** With the patient's arms over her head, the technologist has her slowly lean forward. This causes the breast to become pendulous and move freely away from the chest wall. Once again, the technologist looks for any abnormalities.

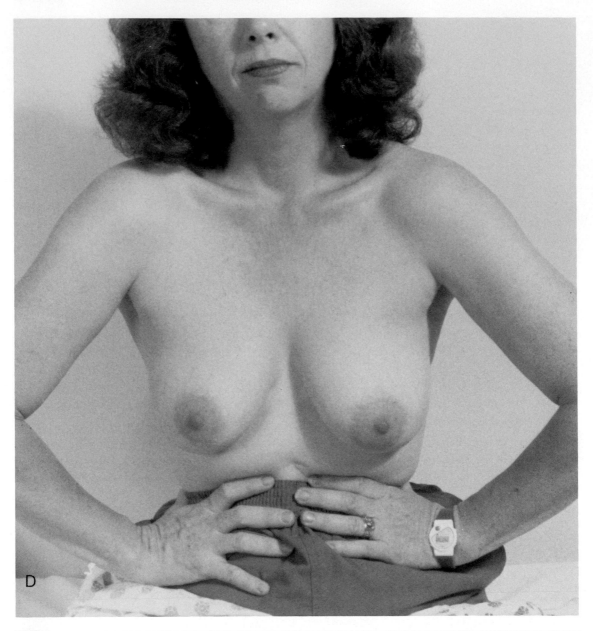

D

Figure 9-2 *Continued.* **D,** Finally, the technologist has the patient place her hands on her hips and press in while contracting her chest muscles.

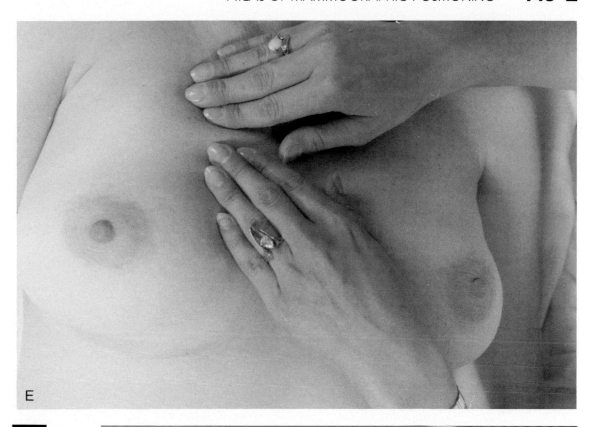

E

Figure 9-2 *Continued.* *E–G,* Positions for a palpation. *E,* The technologist palpates both breasts while the patient is lying down. While the technologist is examining the breast tissue from the nipple to the sternum, the patient may have her arms relaxed at her sides.

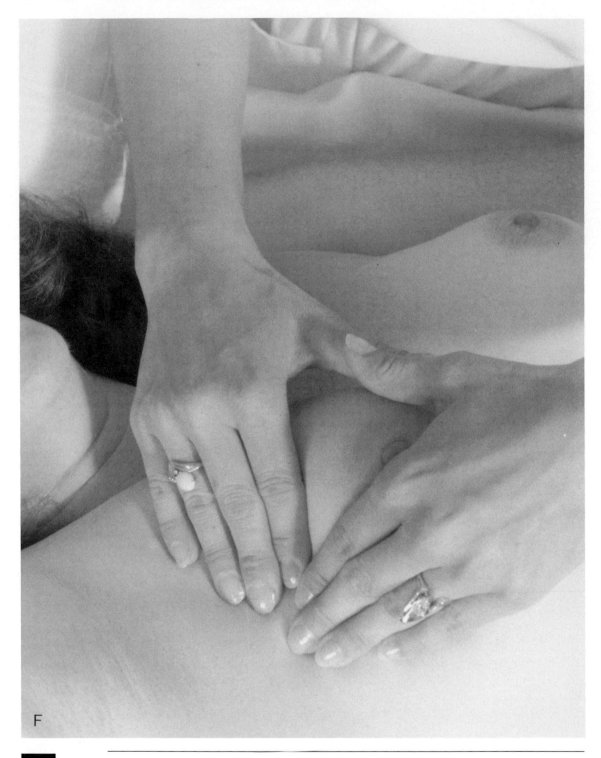

F

Figure 9-2 *Continued.* *F,* For examining breast tissue from the nipple to the ax-illa, the patient's arm on the side of the breast being examined should be bent at a 90° angle with the elbow flexed. If the patient has large breasts, it may be helpful for the technologist to place a sponge or rolled towel under the patient's back on the side of the breast being examined. This will cause the lateral border of the breast to roll medially over the ribs for easier palpation.

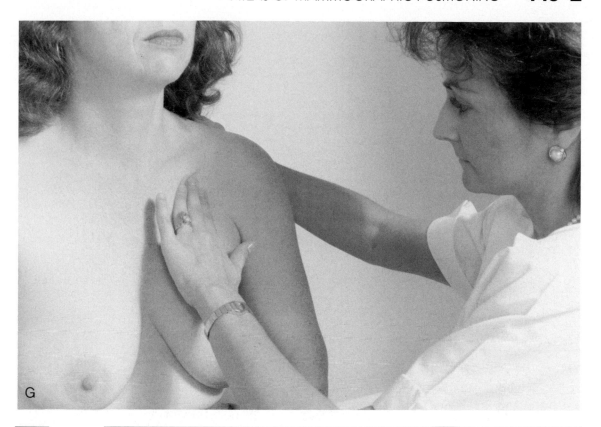

Figure 9-2 *Continued.* **G,** The sitting position is useful for palpating the regional lymph nodes above and below the clavicle.

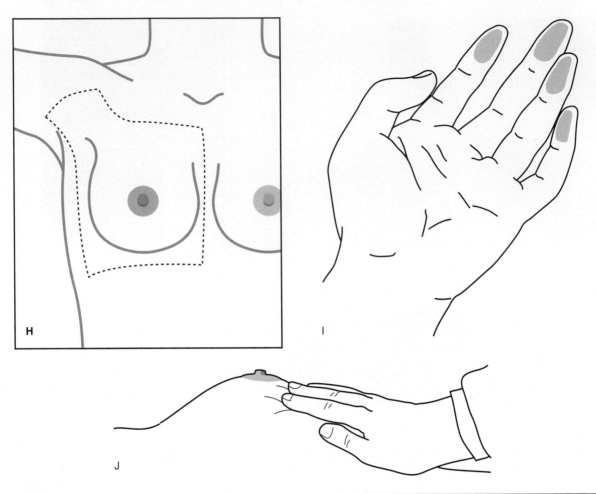

Figure 9-2 *Continued*. *H*, **Perimeter.** All breast tissue should be included in the perimeter of the area to be examined. This perimeter is indicated by the broken line extending vertically from the middle of the axilla to the rib just beneath the breast and continuing horizontally along the bra line or underside of the breast to midsternum. It continues up the sternum to the clavicle, along the lower border of the clavicle to the shoulder, and back to the middle of the axilla.

I, The technologist should use the soft pads of her fingers (shaded area) for the **palpation technique**. Compressing breast tissue with the pads of 3 or 4 of the fingers, the technologist moves the fingers in a dime-sized circular motion. If an abnormality, either a mass or a thickening, is found, the technologist compresses the skin on both sides of the abnormality to flatten or dimple the skin.

J, Abnormalities may be superficial or deep. Varying the level of **pressure** from the pads of the fingers pressing into the breast enables the technologist to find them all. Light pressure may be used to locate superficial abnormalities, and firm pressure can be used to locate abnormalities on the chest wall. If a thickening is felt, a bimanual examination may be helpful to further characterize it.

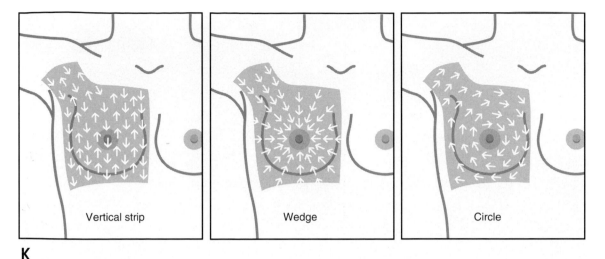

K

Figure 9-2 *Continued.* *K,* **Patterns of search.** It is important to examine all of the breast tissue within the perimeter with a systematic approach. The three patterns that may be used include 1) the vertical strip; 2) the wedge; and 3) the circle. The vertical strip is the most popular pattern used. To perform a clinical breast examination using the vertical strip method, the technologist begins palpating in dime-sized circles at the patient's armpit and proceeding down until reaching the lower boundary or bra line. The technologist moves a finger's width medially and continues palpating back up the breast until reaching the upper boundary. Once again, the technologist moves a finger's width medially and continues downward. The technologist repeats this pattern until all of the breast tissue has been covered to the middle to the sternum. The examination requires from 10 to 16 vertical strips to search each breast.

For the wedge pattern, imagine that the breast is divided as with the spokes of a wheel. The technologist examines each segment of the wheel individually by moving her fingers from the outside boundary in toward the nipple. The technologist then slides her fingers back to the boundary line and moves over a finger's width. The technologist repeats this pattern until the entire breast has been covered. Once again, between 10 and 16 segments of the wedge pattern are needed to search each breast.

For the circle pattern, imagine the breast as the face of a clock. Starting at 12 o'clock, the technologist palpates along the boundary of the outer face of the clock until returning to the starting point. The technologist then moves down a finger's width and continues palpating in even smaller circles until reaching the nipple. Depending on the size of the breast being examined, the technologist will use between 8 and 10 circles to search each breast.

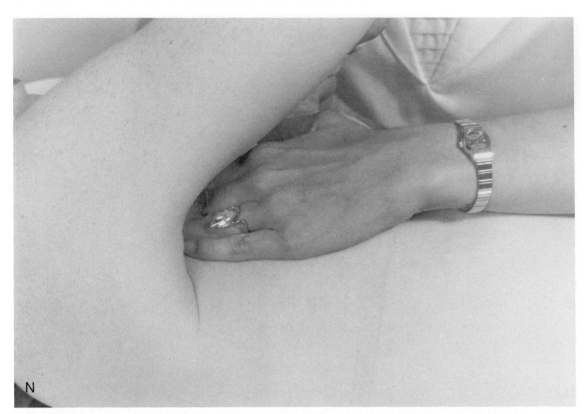

N

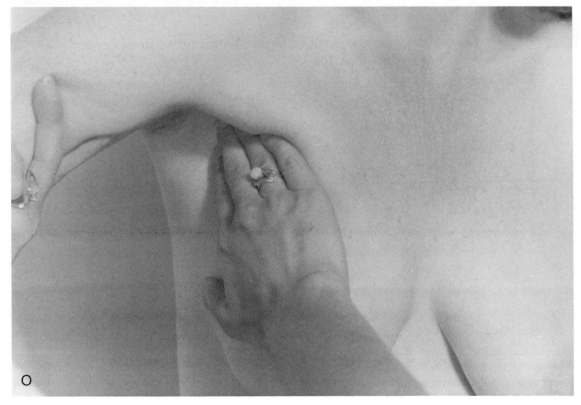

O

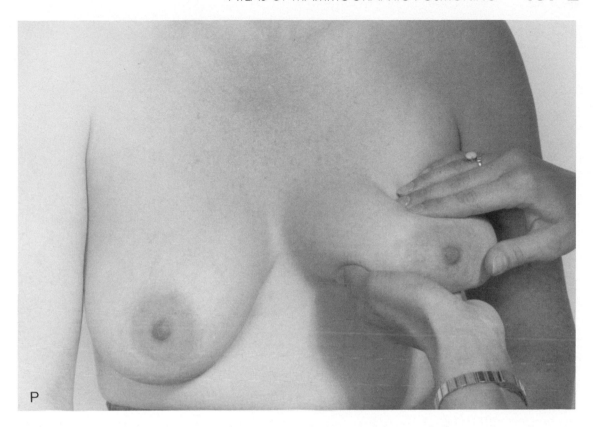

P

Figure 9-2 *Continued.* **N, O,** *Facing page.* A regional lymph node examination should be done with the patient in the supine and upright positions. The technologist should firmly hold the patient's arm on the side of the axilla to be examined so that the patient may keep her pectoral muscle relaxed.

P, *Above.* **Practice with feedback.** Technologists just beginning clinical breast examinations should spend time and perfect their technique with a clinician or radiologist. This will ensure competence and self-confidence. Many facilities encourage their technologists to teach individualized skill-oriented breast self-examination (BSE) to their patients. There are many breast models available today that simulate normal and abnormal characteristics. These may be useful in helping the patient develop her own technique for breast self-examination. Patients should be encouraged to perform breast self-examinations monthly because breast self-examination is a woman's first line of defense against breast cancer.

The plan of action. Each patient should have a personal breast health plan of action. Breast self-examination is only one of three necessary steps in the early detection of breast cancer. Breast self-examination is most effective when combined with mammography and clinical breast examination as outlined in the following American Cancer Society guidelines. Breast self-examination should begin with women at age 20 and be practiced every month. Clinical breast examinations should be performed every 3 years on women between 20 and 40 years old and every year on women over 40 years old. Mammography should be performed every 1 or 2 years on women between 40 and 49 years old. For those patients 50 years old and over, mammography should be performed every year.

CHAPTER TEN

Integrity of the Mammographic Image

Bob Meisch

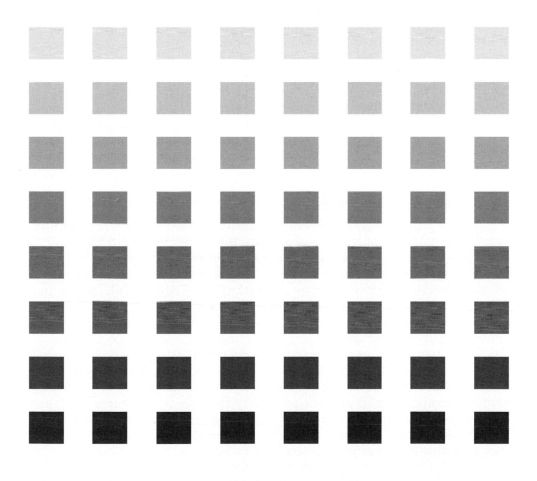

Every book, newsletter, and commercial data sheet, and most other published materials on the subject of mammography, discuss quality control (QC). Most include information on what should be done for processor control.

Important questions are why the technologist should perform processor control a particular way and, even more importantly, what the technologist should do when something goes wrong with the processor. This chapter covers the typical problems with the processor and the steps that are often taken to attempt corrective action. When a service engineer corrects a problem with the equipment, the technologist should ask about the procedure. The more the technologist knows about the reasons for the way to perform QC, the better the quality of his or her mammograms will be. This chapter will not describe the way to do QC, but will address what goes wrong with mammographic films and why. I will first discuss the reasons for problems with mammographic films.

VARIABLES IN FILM PROCESSING

Film manufacturing is an art as well as a science. Inherent variables exist in every emulsion. Chemistry mixing has many variables. Chemical usage and volume turnover, oxidation, and replenishment are factors in QC. Procedural differences in QC from day to day or from person to person create variables. Test equipment changes may also mimic processing changes. Considering also the variables of the patient's size, age, tissue density, compression differences, generating equipment differences, and more, one wonders how film mammography works as well as it does. The reason for QC becomes obvious: to minimize the variables that can be controlled.

The variables most easily controlled are in the processing environment. The following information may vary somewhat from manufacturer to manufacturer but applies to most film processing variables.

Film Speed and Contrast

A processor control graph produced by the technologist shows a drop in film speed and contrast that appears at or below the low limit (Fig. 10-1A).

There is often some question about whether to call the service company. For this example, assume that the service company has been called. The local processor service engineer arrives and makes some adjustment, checks the developer temperature, and drains and refills the developer tank. The service engineer processes a follow-up control strip (Fig. 10-1B), and the processor is almost back in working order.

The action taken in this example is characteristic of the technologist's reaction to problems with mammography processing. We are not sure what went wrong in the equipment or what was done to correct it. If this same problem occurs again, there is a possibility that the same course of action (i.e., the service company's being called) could be taken.

The technologist should see if the clinical images look bad. If the images look all right, it is possible that nothing is wrong with the equipment and that to call the service company would just waste everyone's money and cause unnecessary disposal of seasoned developer. (I will discuss "seasoned" developer later in this chapter.) If something was wrong with the equipment, the chances are that the service engineer could not accurately analyze what it was because of a lack of technical training.

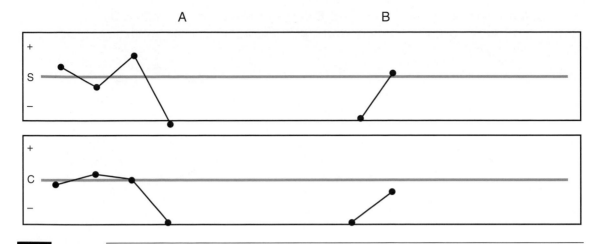

Figure 10-1. *A*, A processor control graph showing a drop in (the film speed (S) and contrast (C). Speed = medium density; contrast = density difference. *B*, The graph obtained after adjustment of the processor by the service engineer.

Developer Temperature

Many new-generation processors maintain tight control of the developer temperature. Older units still in service or rebuilt older units, however, may allow the developer temperature to drift as much as ±2°F. That 4° spread could alter contrast and density by as much as 20 percent, depending on the type of mammography film used. The technologist should never rely on the processor temperature gauge alone; someone may have adjusted the gauge needle. The technologist should always use a high-quality photographic analog or digital thermometer placed directly in the developer tank with the recirculation pump running (out of standby control).

Unless otherwise specified by the manufacturer, the most frequently used temperatures are 95°F for a 90-second cycle and 92°F for a 2- to 2.5-minute cycle (this is not extended). A 5° loss of temperature from normal would require approximately a 25 percent to 30 percent increase in exposure, depending on the film's characteristics. If the developer is hotter than normal after the required warm-up period, there is most likely an electromechanical problem, and service must be called; however; the technologist should always check to ensure that incoming water is running to the processor.

Note: As the temperature increases, the film speed and the contrast increase to a point.

Extremely high temperatures will cause a loss of contrast as the film speed increases and fog begins to increase. *The technologist must always check the developer temperature* (Fig. 10-2A, B, and C).

The developer temperature changes for the following reasons:

1. An incorrect incoming water temperature on older processors requires a mixing valve—the technologist should check the incoming water.

2. The airflow on newer air-cooled processors is restricted—the technologist should check the air intake filter.

3. The heating element fails or is incorrectly adjusted.

4. The recirculation pump fails.

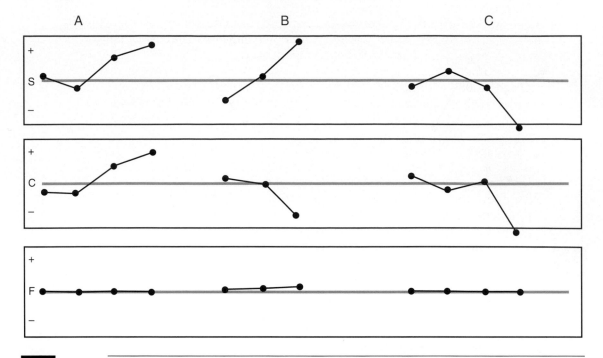

Figure 10-2. Processor control graphs showing the effects of the changes in the developer temperature.

A, The speed (S) and the contrast (C) increase and the fog (F) remains unchanged. The developer temperature is slightly higher than normal. **B**, The speed increases, the fog increases, and the contrast decreases. The developer temperature is excessively high. **C**, The speed and the contrast are both very low with no change in the fog. The developer is probably not up to the operating temperature. Note: Exposing a single-emulsion film backwards will create the same extreme drop on a graph. If this type of change occurs immediately following a processor servicing or chemical change, the technologist should check the specific gravity for overdilution or call the service engineer back immediately.

Developer and Replenisher Dilution

The developer must be mixed to the proper specific gravity (SG). The specific gravity may be measured using an inexpensive hydrometer float. A quality service organization gives its engineers this tool.

Measuring the specific gravity and verifying its accuracy should be done at every processor preventive maintenance interval. This is the only way to ensure proper processor contrast and speed. Using the film manufacturer's chemistry is also a good choice. The technologist should ask the service organization to verify the specific gravity at the mammographic processing site each time the processor is cleaned.

The service engineer needs to compare the specific gravity of a developer with the specific gravity (weight) of water, which is 1.000. A specific gravity of a chemical higher than 1.000 is heavier than water; the value of the specific gravity indicates whether the chemical is overdiluted or underdiluted compared with water.

For example, fresh developer with specific gravity of 1.085 ± 0.0025 in the chemical mixing or holding tank should be normal. An actual reading of

1.079 indicates that the chemical's weight is closer to water's than it should be (i.e., it is overdiluted). A reading of 1.094 indicates that the chemical is overconcentrated, i.e., there is not enough water.

Assume that the specific gravity in the replenisher tank or chemical mixer is 1.087 (acceptable) but the specific gravity in the processor tank is 1.091, which is higher than normal. If the replenisher tank SG is satisfactory at 1.087, and the replenisher tank supplies the processor tank (SG 1.091), how is it possible that the specific gravity is high (overconcentrated) at 1.091 in the processor tank? In fact, this concentration level could be normal. The processor, unlike the replenisher system, is always running in a heated environment that increases evaporation, causing the specific gravity to be slightly higher than normal (i.e., overconcentrated) in the processor while the replenisher tank is normal.

Note: If the developer temperature and the specific gravity are within the manufacturer's specifications and the developer is fairly fresh (5 days old or less) the processor should be running normally. If there is an imaging problem, the problem is probably not in the processor. The technologist must always check or have someone check the chemical's SG when the chemicals are delivered.

Freshly mixed developer replenisher will have a different specific gravity than that of seasoned developer. The technologist should always check the manufacturer's specifications for fresh and seasoned solutions.

Developer Dilution and Evaporation

See Figure 10-3*A* and *B* for a processor control graph showing the effects of developer dilution and evaporation.

Developer and Replenisher Age

The age of mixed developer is also very important. In concentrated form and in separate bottles of parts A, B, and C, the chemicals used to make a developer will usually last approximately 1 year. Once mixed with water, the chemicals become working developer and begin to break down immediately. For this reason, it is very important to ensure that the supplier of the chemicals is mixing and delivering the chemicals often and that the chemical product is not several days old.

The department should store the smallest quantity of mixed (working-strength) solution that is possible. Every 5-gallon unit of chemicals should be turned over in 4 to 5 days maximum or discarded. A chemical supplier must not be allowed to store extra pre-mix on the film processing premises.

It is equally important for the imaging department to turn over the chemicals in the replenisher tank quickly. A system using small quantities in small tanks is the best replenisher system if the department is a low- to medium-volume film user. Using the replenisher quickly reduces the chance of poor film quality on the view box (i.e., wasting a few cents of chemicals each week by turning over the chemicals more rapidly will help to improve the quality on the view box).

A flooded replenishment system may be the best solution to chemical breakdown in departments that are low-volume processors (Fig. 10-4). Some dedicated mammography processors have flooded-system capability built into

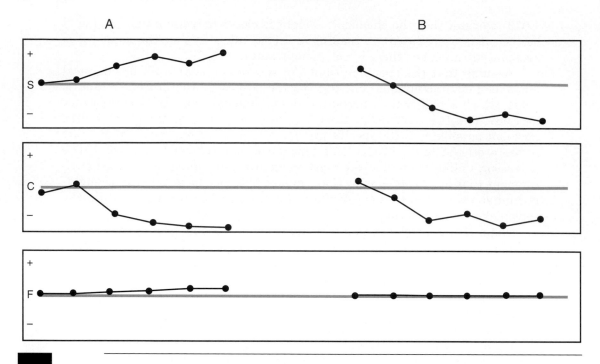

Figure 10-3. Processor control graphs showing the effects of developer dilution and evaporation. ***A***, The speed (S) increases, the contrast (C) decreases, and the fog (F) slightly increases. The developer is overconcentrated or it has evaporated. ***B***, The speed and contrast decrease with no change in the fog. The developer has been overdiluted.

the processor. Others may need a kit for flooded systems; these kits are available from some of the major film manufacturers.

A Case in Point. One might ask why film that looks acceptable when used in main radiology looks bad when used in the operating room (OR). This inconsistency occurs because the chemicals in the OR sit day after day, sometimes week after week, with little or no replenishment. Oxidation starts immediately after chemical mixing. Low volume replenishment and low film usage reduce the chemical turnover, and the film contrast begins to drop dramatically. The restrainer in the developer, along with everything else, breaks down; the film speed increases, fog increases, and the film contrast drops below acceptable limits.

Developer Replenishment

Always follow the film manufacturer's specifications for replenisher based on the film volume and seasoning.

Fixer Temperature and Dilution

Fixer Temperature. Although little attention is given to fixer tempera-

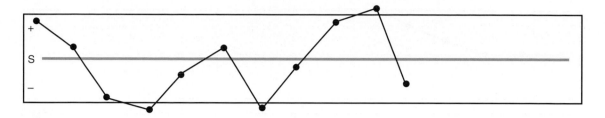

Figure 10-4. A processor control graph showing low-volume processing. The graph shows significant swings in the speed (the contrast also decreases) and is typical of a low-volume processing environment.

ture, it is very important in QC. If the temperature is below normal, the fixer will not properly clear the radiographic films. This is very obvious on single-emulsion films used in mammography; the film appears to have a smoky or hazy nonclearing background. Archival quality is also affected by lower-than-normal fixer temperature.

The largest single cause for nonclearing film if the fixer is correctly diluted is use of a processor that has been *cold-water converted*. The problem may not manifest itself in a warm-weather climate, but in northern American states, especially in winter, the problem can be extreme. This cold-water conversion will also have a negative effect on archival quality.

Older-model processors require mixing valves to maintain the temperature of the water coming into the wash tank at approximately 8° below the developer temperature. The developer recirculates through tubes in the wash tank, thus providing the cooling process for the developer. Normally, the developer tank is at 95°F, and the washwater supplied through the mixing valve is at approximately 87°F, 8° lower than the developer temperature.

The fixer tank sits between the 95° developer tank and the 87° wash tank. The heated developer is slightly cooled by the 87° water. If the mixing valve is removed and the processor converted to "cold water," problems could result. With this change, the incoming washwater in the winter months could be 80°, 70°, 50° or even colder in a northern state.

The fixer is heated by the 95° developer by heat transfer through the walls of the developer to the fix tank. The very cold water in the washwater tank also transfers heat from the fixer to the cold water tank, and the fixer temperature drops. Hence, the films may not clear properly and the archival quality is in jeopardy.

The heat indicator light for the developer on the front of the processor usually works overtime (i.e., runs excessively) under a field-converted situation. In some instances, a slight fixer odor may also be noticed on the films. The warmer the fixer temperature, the better the film will clear.

Fixer Dilution. The fixer dilution is very important. If the fixer is overdiluted, the films will not clear properly. The films may also dry insufficiently and be tacky, causing film jams in the fixer or dryer of a processor. Overconcentration of the fixer is very rare but can be verified by measuring the chemical's specific gravity. Always use the chemical manufacturer's specifications for the specific gravity and have the chemical supply company verify the specific gravity.

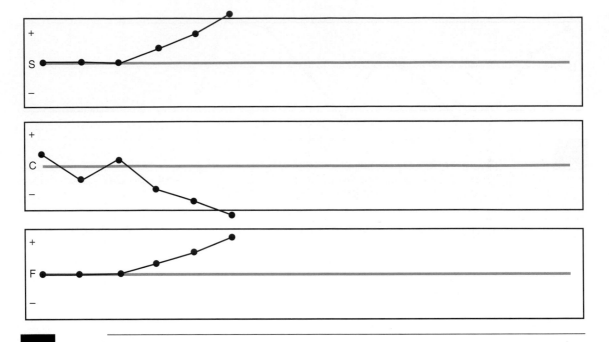

Figure 10-5. A processor control graph showing the effects of developer contamination. (S = speed; C = contrast; F = fog.)

Developer Contamination. When the developer is contaminated, the fog increases (i.e., unexposed silver is being developed) the film speed increases, and the film contrast drops. The developer must be changed (Fig. 10-5).

COMMON EQUIPMENT AND PROCEDURAL ERRORS

Graph interpretation is always a challenge. A "spike" in a graph may indicate not a problem but rather a procedural error (Fig. 10-6A). A trend on the graph does indicate a potential problem (Fig. 10-6B). The technologist should always question,whether the clinical images look all right. If they do, there is a possibility that a procedural error took place or there were slight variations within the test equipment. The technologist should always use the QC equipment in exactly the same manner for each test. Attention to this detail will minimize operator-induced variations in the sensitometric readings. Following are a few examples of common equipment and procedural errors.

Operator-Induced Variations

1. Look at the aperture in the densitometer, located on the surface of the unit where density is measured. Most manufacturers provide with each machine an envelope containing different-sized apertures. A large aperture could allow the reader to accidentally catch two adjacent steps at once and thus read two partial and different densities. The technologist should use the smallest aperture to ensure the measurement of one step at a time.

2. The technologist must make sure the step reading is done in the center of the appropriate step. A reading slightly left or right of center on any step could give a slight change in density from left to right. This change will mimic density variations in the processor.

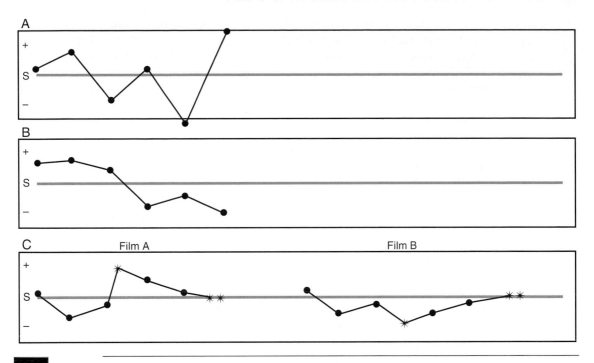

Figure 10-6. *A*, A processor control graph showing a spike, indicating the possibility of a procedural error. ***B***, A processor control graph showing a trend, indicating a processing problem. This trend calls for processor attention. ***C***, A processor control graph comparing fresh (*) and seasoned (**) developer. (S = speed.) (See text page 162.)

3. When in doubt, zero it out! Even if recalibration or rezeroing was done at the initial start-up of the densitometer, it is a good idea to double check the "zero" calibration even after the densitometer warms up.

Density Control. Densitometers are usually shipped with the manufacturer's control density strip. This is a simple density strip with a few known density values already measured and documented. It should be used semiannually to verify the accuracy of the densitometer. The technologist should read the test strip using the department's densitometer and compare the readings to the values marked on the manufacturer's control density strip. If a density difference greater than 0.03 exists between the technologist's reading and the density marked on the control density strip, the technologist should contact the manufacturer for recommendations.

Reproducibility of the Sensitometer. Reproducibility of the sensitometer is also critical. A semiannual check for reproducibility is a good practice. The technologist should take a 14 x 17-inch sheet of film and produce multiple exposures around its perimeter. The technologist should not flip the emulsion over. A delay of approximately 20 seconds between exposures will allow the sensitometer to stabilize. This single sheet of film with many exposed strips on it will eliminate film-sheet to film-sheet and processing variables. The technologist should process the film and read any density step with a density of approximately 1.0 plus gross fog, the speed point for medical x-ray film.

The technologist should read the same step on each exposure around the perimeter of the film. If the density varies significantly from one density strip to another on the same sheet of film, the sensitometer produced different intensities from one exposure to another. The manufacturer should be called for assistance.

Processor Cleaning. Different manufacturers' films (A versus B in Fig. 10-6C) react differently to different starters following a processor cleaning. The technologist should always use the same manufacturer's developer starter solution. Brands should not be intermixed, as the sensitometric exposures may vary. When a processor is cleaned, developer is drained from the processor tank and discarded. All of the seasoning goes with the developer. Starter solution is used to "start" the developer but will not "season" it much beyond the initial first few days following a cleaning. As more film is processed, more seasoning occurs until full seasoning is achieved. In low-volume mammography processing, the processor has the potential (because of the frequency of cleaning) not to reach full seasoning from one cleaning to the next. This has been a problem in surgery suites since the first automatic processor was placed in them.

A simple but effective way to ensure continuous seasoning regardless of the cleaning interval is to have the service representative reserve some of the old developer when the unit is cleaned. Adding approximately 1 gallon of old developer (full of seasoning) to the developer tank along with the remainder of the new developer will provide instant seasoning. This could reduce or even eliminate the QC difference between films processed from seasoned old developer and those processed in fresh new developer each time a processor is cleaned. The normal amount of starter solution should also be used.

Processor Dryer Temperature. The dryer temperature should be set only high enough to fully dry a film. A standard temperature is approximately 125° to 130°. If the processor has sufficient dryer temperature and air circulation, the films will dry. If the film feels wet but the surface appears "hard," it indicates a dryer problem. If the film is wet and it feels "tacky," however, this suggests insufficient fixing. The specific gravity should be checked.

CHAPTER ELEVEN

Mammography Artifacts–
Their Causes and Cures

Bob Meisch

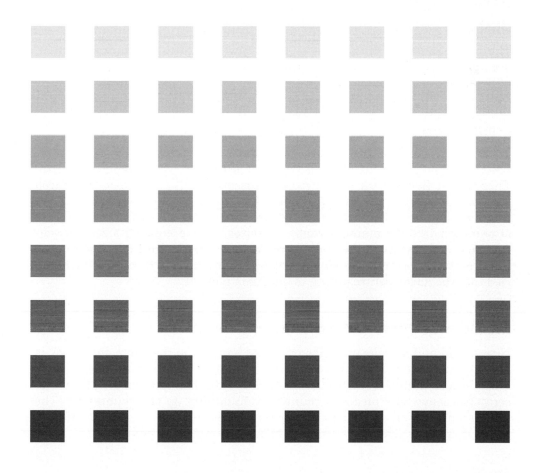

Artifacts are an unwanted but normal part of radiologic imaging and are of great concern in mammography. Mammographic artifacts may be controlled with a small amount of effort. Much is written about quality mammography, but few specifics are available on controlling the very important and ongoing problem of artifacts.

As film sensitometric characteristics have improved, providing greater levels of film contrast and speed, artifact visualization has actually increased. Contrast improvements exaggerate the edges of the artifacts. The single-emulsion films used in all radiographic applications have more potential for artifacts than double-emulsion materials, although the problem is often less obvious in nuclear medicine or ultrasonography, in which single-emulsion technology produces dark images on a clear background. Unlike in nuclear medicine or ultrasound imaging, a dust artifact in mammography may mimic microcalcification in the breast tissue.

The proper identification of imaging or processor-generated artifacts is difficult and can be frustrating. Usually, artifacts that are blamed on the film or the processor are most often caused by other factors.

GENERAL CAUSES

Dust and Dirt

The major causes of 90 percent or more of all artifacts are darkroom dust, dirt, and poor housekeeping habits in and around the processing/film-handling area.

Paint Flakes

Every darkroom that has a passbox in the wall has had microscopic paint flakes scraped off the inside walls from the passage of conventional cassettes. These paint flakes stick to the regular cassettes if the darkroom is shared with mammography processing and are deposited onto the countertops of the film-handling area. Paint flakes can cause three kinds of artifacts. The flakes of paint get into the mammography cassettes, thus producing a screen/radiographic artifact. Also, the flakes are deposited from the film surface onto the processor feed tray, causing scratches. Finally, some flakes are also carried into the developer, resulting in emulsion pick-off.

Multiformat Cassette Scratches and Debris

Ultrasound and nuclear medicine cassettes handled in the same darkroom as for mammography cassettes create another major source of artifacts. Every multiformat camera cassette "darkslide" has scratches from loading film. The scratches leave tiny pieces of paint and aluminum on the countertop. The same artifact "trail" described earlier occurs, resulting in the three different types of artifacts. They all have the potential to mimic pathology.

SPECIFIC CAUSES AND "CURES"

The causes and cures of mammography artifacts are easy to manage with a small amount of effort each day.

Pick-off

"Pick-off" is usually cited by processor service engineers attempting to find the cause of artifacts. Although pick-off may be created within the processor, its real cause is usually foreign material (dust and dirt) from the darkroom film handling area that made its way into the processor.

Pick-off unfortunately is a normal occurrence every time a double- or single-emulsion radiographic film is processed. This is one reason many processors have developer filters to pick up emulsion debris in the developing section of the processor.

Pick-off usually appears as sharp-edged, bright white specks that are randomly distributed across the surface of a film.

Some causes of pick-off include

1. foreign material in the processor
2. a dirty developer filter
3. dried chemicals on the rollers in the developer

To "cure" pick-off,

1. all sections of the processor must be clean
2. the developer filter must be changed every preventive maintenance interval
3. the crossovers should be cleaned each day prior to processing films
4. clean-up films should be run each day or following any long period of standby control.

Pressure-Mottle Positive Density Texture

The causes of a pressure-mottle positive density texture include

1. microscopic scratches and bumps on any soft surface processor roller (most often in the developer rack) caused by using an abrasive type of cleaning pad (e.g., Scotch-Brite)

2. excessive tension on the squeegee rollers, forcing excessive development of the emulsion

3. bad developer rollers

Although an abrasive type of cleaning pad works well, it acts like sandpaper on soft surface processor rollers. After several maintenance cycles, the soft surface rollers begin to show signs of tiny bumps as a result of the "sanding" action. The tiny bumps create excessive development of tiny spots on the mammogram, thus producing pressure mottle or microscopic spots of overdevelopment.

To "cure" this problem, the technologist should require the service company to

1. replace the suspect rollers, especially the 1-inch black plastic roller in the developer rack
2. correct the loss of the hardener in the developer from incorrect dilution, underreplenishment, or oxidized or old developer
3. check the chemical's specific gravity against the manufacturer's specifications; replenisher rates must be set according to the film manufacturer's specifications (if low-volume processing exists, a flooded replenisher system is advised)

Until mixed with water, parts A, B, and C of any chemical concentrate are technically not working developer, but separate and different chemical concentrates. Once mixed, the working developer replenisher begins to deteriorate immediately. Every 5 gallons of diluted developer replenisher should be used in 4 to 5 days. Small tanks should be used and turned over quickly.

The technologist should not store extra premixed jugs of developer. Although this may benefit the chemistry supplier, the old chemicals can ruin the clinic's mammograms (through oxidation).

The technologist should *use solid one-piece floating lids,* never small individual floating balls or stars, for an evaporation cover. Balls are unacceptable because no one removes them before refilling the replenisher tanks; as a result, oxidized developer on the small float surfaces is rinsed into the working tank when it is refilled.

Surface Scratches

The causes of surface scratches include

1. incoming water impurities
2. emulsion fed "down"

To "cure" surface scratches,

1. the mammography processor must have a water filter on the incoming water line with a *No by-pass* feature
2. the technologist should feed the emulsion "up"
3. the technologist should clean the processor feed tray daily

White Specks

White specks include pick-off, screen artifacts, and radiographic artifacts. This is the biggest group of problem artifacts and the easiest to cure.

The causes of white specks include

1. darkroom dust
2. dirt
3. poor housecleaning habits in the processing area and countertop dust and dirt on the shelf just above the film countertop (where the extra film boxes or the technologist's personal belongings are stored)

To "cure" white specks, the technologist should

1. damp and dry-wipe film handling areas daily
2. check the ceiling ventilator, which may be full of dust and soot
3. clean the shelves over the countertops
4. wipe out any passboxes daily
5. check all non-mammography cassettes for chips or debris if they are used in the same darkroom as for mammography cassettes
6. clean the processor feed tray daily
7. most importantly, the facility should replace any "suspended ceiling" with a solid drywalled ceiling; otherwise, the suspended ceiling panels will move slightly every time the darkroom door is opened and closed, allowing tiny dust specks from the ceiling to fall onto the countertop, into the cassettes, on the processor feed tray, and into the processor

Restrictive Development

Restrictive development causes a negative density artifact, usually running parallel to the rollers. This artifact may resemble waves on the ocean owing to the liquid motion of the developer tank. It may also mimic pick-off.

Antistatic coating on certain films causes restrictive development.

This coating, which is insoluble, could be suspended on the surface of the developer. This action is similar to that of oil on water. As a film passes through the developer, the antistatic coating can stick to the surface of the film, causing less than full development in that area of the x-ray film.

Complete processor cleaning during preventive maintenance is critical. The service company should not cut corners on maintenance in this area. All racks, rollers, tanks, filters, and recirculation lines and tubing must be completely flushed and cleaned.

Runback

Runback is defined as positive density streaks on the trailing edge of the radiograph.

The causes of runback include

1. improper squeegee roller tension
2. a worn squeegee roller

To "cure" runback, the service company should

1. correct alignment problems with the squeegee rollers
2. replace worn squeegee rollers
3. make sure that squeegee and crossover rollers are free floating, not frozen or stuck

Stub Line

A stub line is a positive density "line" artifact running parallel to the rollers of a rack at approximately 1-5/8 inch from the leading edge of a film.

Stub lines are caused by the film's "stubbing" against a turnaround roller or guide shoe of a rack, causing a momentary stall of the film transport. A developer roller spins on the surface of the film, causing excessive film development in the form of a positive density line.

To "cure" stub line artifacts, the service company should

1. correct the adjustment of the guide shoe if it is adjustable
2. feed the emulsion "up" the film curls in the direction of the turnaround rollers, not against it
3. *in extreme cases* on X-OMAT units, replace the bottom roller (see Eastman Kodak service bulletin number 87)

Static Discharge

Static discharge causes positive density artifacts: random "tree, lightning, dot" artifacts.

The cause of static discharge is low humidity, typical of a cold weather climate during the heating season.

To "cure" static discharge, the technologist should add humidity to the processing environment—approximately 50 percent or greater humidity is needed.

Milky Appearance

The causes of a milky appearance include

1. cold fixer
2. overdiluted fixer
3. severely underreplenished fixer

To "cure" a milky appearance, the fixer temperature should be close to the developer temperature. The technologist should avoid "converted cold water" processors—if the manufacturer did not build it cold-water compatible, the technologist should not buy it.

The fixer temperature in a cold climate could be affected by this type of conversion unit, thus causing improper film clearing.

The technologist should

1. verify the specific gravity of the fixer and replace it if needed
2. check the replenisher rates for the film volume
3. check for a kinked replenisher line

Radiographic Artifacts

Radiographic artifacts can be caused by any object in the "image in space" path. These include manufacturing machining "chips" inside the collimeter, bucky texture, or damaged or defective grids. When all other artifacts are eliminated, the service company should contact the original manufacturer of the radiographic equipment for assistance.

Bibliography

1. American Cancer Society of California: Clinical Breast Examination: Proficiency Criteria and Guidelines, 1989.
2. American College of Radiology: 25th National Conference on Breast Cancer Course Syllabus. Boston, MA, 1992.
3. American College of Radiology: Train the Trainer Seminar Course Syllabus. Reston, VA, 1992.
4. Basset L: Breast imaging—current status and future directions. Radiol Clin North Am 30(1):21–53, 139–153, 1992.
5. General Electric Medical Systems: Mammography Positioning Workshop for Application Specialists Course Syllabus. Milwaukee, WI, 1991.
6. Homer M: Mammographic Interpretation: A Practical Approach. New York, McGraw-Hill, 1991, pp. 4–15, 30–58, 59–70, 74–99, 112–113, 114–139.
7. Komen SG: The Breast Imaging Seminar Course Syllabus. Peoria, IL, 1991.
8. Kopans D: Breast Imaging. Philadelphia, J.B. Lippincott, 1989, pp. 34–114, 320–337, 342–350.
9. Long S: Handbook of Mammography, 1990.
10. Medical Technology Management Institute: Mammography Course for Technologists Course Syllabus, 1991 and 1992.

INDEX

Note: Page numbers in *italics* indicate illustrations; page numbers followed by t indicate tables.